CW00590486

META **Messages**
from Your Body

Discover the **Cause** of Disease and Why Your Body Doesn't Make **Mistakes**

B Y   S A M   T H O R P E

www.TheSuccessfulAuthor.com

Foreword

by Karl Dawson

I am delighted to write the foreword to this book. I have personally been involved with META-Health (the new name for META-Medicine worldwide) for some years. As one of the original Emotional Freedom Techniques (EFT) Masters, I have benefited from the wisdom and understanding of such great teachers as Gary Craig, Donna Gates, cellular biologist Dr Bruce Lipton and trauma expert Dr Robert Scaer. In the course of my learning and practice, I have come to appreciate the ways in which the body and mind are inextricably linked to our patterns of illness. As Sam Thorpe points out in her thoughtful introduction,

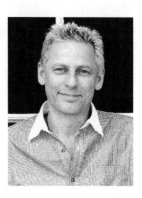

Karl Dawson, EFT Master and creator of Matrix Reimprinting using EFT

META-Health provides a missing link between our past experiences and beliefs and the diseases that come to us.

I've always found it amazing how little modern medicine is able to tell us about the origins of the vast majority of diseases, despite the very precise diagnosis that it can offer of the exact type of dysfunction within the body, be it genetic, chemical, hormonal, cellular or some invading organism. Yet, when it comes to the cause of the disease there is so often the answer – unknown!!

Many diseases are put simply down to 'stress' as a catch-all term for many conditions where the causation is unclear. But what exactly is stress and how can it cause such a myriad of health problems?

The exciting science of epigenetics gives a strong indication of how stress creates illness. It is not so much the inner workings of the cell that predisposes us to certain diseases, but rather the way in which we interact with our surroundings.

As the subtitle of Sam's book suggests, disease is not an accident. So-called emotional and physical diseases are the body's attempt to make physiological changes to be better able to deal with the life situations that we face.
What makes us behave in a certain way in any given situation? Whether our reactions are positive or negative, it is our previous life experiences that determine our responses. When experiencing traumatic events we create beliefs and reach decisions about ourselves and the world. These assumptions go straight into our subconscious minds and become templates as to how we will react in similar, future situations.

So what are these beliefs? They create perceptions such as 'I'm alone', 'People don't like me', 'The world's a dangerous place', 'I'm stupid', 'Whatever I do, it's never good enough', 'I need to be in control', 'I need to be perfect' and an endless array of other misperceptions.

As our negative beliefs interact with our lives, we are led to respond with a degree of fear, frequently expressed as the 'fight or flight' reaction. This is the state of stress that changes every bodily system and function. When we live in this state on a regular basis, our bodies will start to make changes on a cellular, chemical and hormonal level. Even our genetic readout can be affected by this state.

In this fascinating book, you'll see how our different perceptions affect different bodily systems and organs. Armed with a medical diagnosis from your doctor, you'll learn how these negative perceptions can be identified and then resolved to relieve your stress and allow your body to heal.

It is noticeable how many professional therapists came to their understanding through struggle with their own issues. In this book, Sam describes with typical frankness her path from the dark night of the soul back to light and health. In a similar way, my introduction to energy therapies also began with my own illness. Since I began my own journey to health in 2001, I have found META-Health to be an invaluable tool in helping me to make sense of my own conditions, which have included chronic fatigue, multiple allergies, inflammation, metabolic imbalance and severe pain.

It was as a result of my direct personal experience of illness and recovery that I went on to develop an advancement of EFT that has become known worldwide as Matrix Reimprinting. This powerful technique combines quantum physics and the new sciences in a methodology that enables you to work with awareness of your earlier self, as well as to interact directly with the events of that time to alter your beliefs and to learn the lessons from your experiences.

Since a professional META-Health analysis can pinpoint the type and timing of the event that specifically leads to one's illness, it is a natural fit with Matrix Reimprinting. Using the investigative power of META-Health to track down the past trauma, you can resolve its associated stress and impacts on your present health and wellbeing with Matrix Reimprinting.

This information is invaluable whether you are a psychiatrist, psychologist, counsellor, cognitive behavioural therapist, hypnotherapist or follow any other discipline where being able quickly and accurately to uncover underlying negative beliefs and traumas is a key part of your therapy. It is equally accessible if you are a layperson who just wants to understand and resolve the reasons why you are sick.

I have known Sam for several years. Indeed, she credits me in this book with starting her on her path out of the abyss and on to the road towards her mastery of many key energy therapies. I now invite Sam to many of my courses, where she shares her amazing knowledge and introduces the concepts of META-Health in order to help my participants to make these links for themselves and their clients and to understand their own underlying issues.

Sam is a genius at this work: I know the best META-Health people in the world and have been exposed to its concepts myself for over seven years. Sam is one of my main sources of knowledge on META-Health. Her depth of understanding and her ability to simplify and to make accessible what is sometimes complex information is amazing. This probably has much to do with her background as a teacher. She is an excellent presenter and has spoken at some of the biggest EFT events in Europe.

These presentational skills shine through in this book. It is written in an informal style that will appeal to the interested professional or layperson alike, anxious to discover why life seems to have dealt them a bad hand and how they can come to grips with their own healing.

At the same time, it is firmly grounded in the most recent evidence-based research in the field and will be able to stand unapologetically alongside other professional literature on the subject. I expect this book to become a standard introduction to the topic of META-Health and to bring many more people to an understanding of their personal power to maintain and to recover their own health.

Dedication

There are two people in my life without whom I would not be the success I am today.

I dedicate this book to my mum, Ann Pritchard, who gave and continues to give me all a child could ever need and whose truly unconditional love continues to demonstrate to me that love has no boundaries.

I also dedicate this book to my husband, Vic Thorpe. He is a man whose heart is as big as the universe and whose indefatigable dedication to helping and empowering the oppressed and disenfranchised of the world has done more to change the global workplace than he will ever comprehend in his lifetime.

What both Vic and my mum have in common is that they love far beyond their comprehension and capacity with no expectation and no conditions.

I am so privileged to have this life and to have their love.

Mum and Vic, I offer the merits of this book to both of you and also to those that have never been fortunate to know the kind of love that you have gifted to me. I do this with a depth of gratitude that can only be expressed in the Huna prayer of *Ho'oponopono*;

I am sorry, please forgive me, I love you, thank you.

Sam

Acknowledgements

My first acknowledgement must, without a doubt, go to my husband, Vic Thorpe. Little did I know, when I took on the project of writing this book, how much work *he* would have to do! He has been my primary editor, sounding board and support all the way through.

Without the kindness and belief of Karl Dawson I may not even have been here today. Karl gave me a chance when I was at my lowest and the day I met him saved my life. I am grateful to Karl for that chance to turn my life around and for the best introduction to EFT, META-Health[1] and Matrix Reimprinting that I could ever have.

I have had the greatest fortune to be gifted the most outstanding trainers and Rob van Overbruggen comes at the top of that list. Not only does Rob have the depth of knowledge and expertise that makes him one of the leading authorities in META-Health, he also is gentle, fun and endearing. I take great pride in learning from him as a health coach, a trainer and as a thoughtful, respectful role model.

I would like to say 'thank you' to all my clients and students for making my job so rewarding. I am grateful to those who have allowed me to use their cases throughout the book; even if I have changed the names, I appreciate your candour in allowing me to share your stories.

I must give special thanks also to Johannes R. Fisslinger for his great passion and pursuit in sharing META-Health with the world. I owe great gratitude to both Johannes and Dr Anton Bader, without whom we would not have the International META-Medicine Association.

---

1. META-Medicine and META-Health are registered trademarks of the International META-Medicine Association.

My book coach, Kevin Bermingham, has been a gentle but firm guide who insisted that I stuck to my plan and trusted his process. It still amazes me that I have created this book in such a short time. This is a testament to Kevin's expertise and to his highly effective writing programme.

I must thank my proofreaders for following me in such an intense programme. A very special thanks must go to my friends and colleagues, Claire Ballantyne and Eleanor Hatherley. Claire has dedicated much time and effort to editing and offering suggestions with a view to making the book clearer and more concise for translation. I had no idea when I asked Eleanor to proofread the manuscript that she used to be a professional proofreader; her attention to detail really pulled the book together at the end. A special mention is due also of two dear friends and colleagues, who helped me to push through when my personal stuff came up as a result of writing this book. Thank you, Kate Marillat and Sandra Hillawi for your support and expertise.

I would also like to give a special thank you to my colleague and fellow Master Trainer, Penny Croal. Penny continues to be a shining example both personally and professionally. She has integrity, honesty and expertise that make me proud to work alongside her.

Finally, I would like to offer a special thanks to my graphic designers: Mike Beales, who has worked closely with me to produce the front cover and the amazing graphics throughout the book, and Vincent Sneed, who specially designed my four bunnies for me. They really bring the book to life!

Sam Thorpe
Brighton, August 2013

Contents

Introduction

*"Yesterday I was clever, so I wanted to change the world.
Today I am wise, so I am changing myself."* **Rumi**[2]

I have something to share. I have exciting and life-changing information that will change the way you will see your health, and ultimately your everyday life, forever.

> *What you are about to read in this book has the potential to change you from passive bystander to active creator in your own life."*

I believe that once you have learned this information it will be hard to go back. Whether you will have the impetus to act upon it is, of course, up to you. What you are about to read in this book has the potential to change you from passive bystander to active creator in your own life.

My wish is to share with you how this information has changed my life and in turn to open the same opportunities to you. I am driven by a desire to evoke the same 'Aha!' moment in you as I have experienced myself and as I see in my clients and students every day. That unique moment when the connection is made and the pieces of the puzzle all fit into place. Those 'Aha!' moments are equally as profound for me as they are for those whom I work with. I am constantly in awe of how incredible we are as human beings – how highly intuitive, intelligent and adaptive.

This book is aimed at those who are ready to update their map of the world, to navigate new territory and to revisit the old territory with fresh eyes.

---

2. *The Essential Rumi – New Expanded Edition*, Jalal al-Din Rumi, translated by Coleman Barks with John Moyne, HarperSanFrancisco, New York, 2004

1

It is for those that want to have a more active role in their own health. These pages will encourage you to take off the blinkers that have prevented you from seeing yourself in your totality, your completeness and, yes – your awesomeness. It is not my mission to convince people who are not ready to view the world and their health in a different way. If you are looking for confirmation that your existing reality is the only reality, then this book will be somewhat of a strain for you, because it offers possibilities that shift the foundation of what most of us have commonly accepted as 'reality'. If, on the other hand, you feel that you should have more influence over your health, wealth and happiness, or if you feel frustrated and dissatisfied with your current health situation, you need look no further - this book is for you. If you are daunted by the prospect of spending the rest of your life managing symptoms, the information in these pages will be a candle in the darkness. It can shed light on the bigger picture and enable you to step towards new horizons and new opportunities for growth and health.

In the course of this book, I will guide you through some remarkable discoveries and discuss with you the impact that this has on our existing model of health, as well as on our view of each other and the world.

What if...?

I encourage you to read this book with an open and enquiring mind. Ask yourself the question 'What if...?' All the principles that have been drawn together and presented here are backed by scientific research and experiential evidence. Such evidence is freely available in the public domain and if you require this kind of proof to entertain such new and radical concepts, I encourage you to search further for yourself. You will find plenty of information and I give some suggested reading both in the footnotes in the text and in the Resources section at the back of this book. I offer here only my personal view of how this information has been of use to me. I can speak with authority about my own personal experience and what I have learned from my own illnesses. I will share with you my own health issues and how they became the key to my physical, mental and emotional health as well as to my personal and spiritual growth. Often I have used client case studies to demonstrate more complex health problems.

This book is an introduction to the concepts and models of META-Health and is not an individual diagnostic tool in itself. Neither is it a directory of illnesses and their META meanings. However, you will find examples and case studies throughout that demonstrate the connections and META meanings of many common physical and psychological illnesses. There is also a section that will enable you to begin to make sense of your own illness, by analysing your symptoms using META principles (See *The META-Health analysis*, Chapter 5.) You will learn what aspects of your life you need to start paying attention to that will help you to join the dots to form your own picture for health. If you are able to take such a new viewpoint, you will be left in no doubt as to how your body responds to your thoughts and the world around you. You will see for yourself why the body does not make mistakes, but is actually helping you to resolve your life issues.

All case studies included in this book are based on real people; however, the best evidence beyond any shadow of a doubt is that which you experience for yourself. This book is primarily for you, the reader who wants to make connections and make sense of the messages your body is giving you, so that you can understand what you can do to grow and heal. This is the start of your own journey to reconnect with yourself.

What do I know?

The journey I took to get to where I am now was not a pretty one and there were times when I nearly gave up.

One of the greatest fears of suffering from an illness like depression or chronic fatigue is that you will return to the depths of the dark pit of despair that you have been in. Whenever I had some respite from my depression or fatigue, I would try to make the most of the energy I had, in order to 'catch up' again. This inevitably led to a sense of being overwhelmed and so to another relapse. This is a vicious cycle for many people suffering from these illnesses. It felt as if I would never truly be free of that dark cloud, once I had made its acquaintance. That was until I found energy therapies and META-Medicine (which we now call META-Health).

I feel I must preface this book with an explanation about my upbringing. I will talk about early childhood traumas and use examples of my own experiences, when I formed limiting beliefs and made decisions that affected my life. I must explain that I was very lucky to have had the most loving and supportive family - especially my mother, Ann. There has never been a day when she faltered in her love and support. I am so deeply indebted to her for the loving, creative and expressive childhood her love afforded me. What I hope to demonstrate by using examples from my own childhood is how the simplest and most innocuous events can lead us to form very powerful decisions about the world and about ourselves. I had a very happy childhood and yet began to struggle through my teenage years with feeling increasingly misunderstood and unheard. I developed lower-back problems after an incident when, as a joke, someone pulled a chair out as I went to sit down. In my twenties, I became depressed about a relationship and, after giving up my teaching job, began to suffer with chronic fatigue. I seemed unable to control the world around me, to have what I desired and to be happy.

When I look back at photos of myself, I feel that I have been different people at different times. I am not sure if this was because of a struggle to find my identity or a need to explore my identity. Perhaps they are one and the same. Those who know me will testify that I certainly don't do things by halves, which is interesting when I consider that my whole life has been spent trying to avoid being pigeonholed and defined in any specific way. You could say that I went out of my way to remain undefined. I define myself as indefinable.

There are many ways to express your individuality. Those who struggle to define themselves may explore different routes. I expressed myself through my body. I claimed and celebrated my individuality with tattoos and piercings and, in 2000, I saw in the millennium by beginning hormone treatment and surgery for gender reassignment. Not to be a man, but to be androgynous – gender neutral.

Transcending gender

Just before I embarked upon this part of my journey I was ordained a Lay Buddhist of the Order of Buddhist Contemplatives (Soto Zen). I used to spend a lot of time at the Telford Buddhist Priory and most weekends I would assist Reverend Alexander, the Prior. I remember speaking to him about my thoughts and feelings and I ended by saying, 'I am not sure that makes any sense.' To which he replied, 'Oh yes, it is like transcending gender.' I still find this the perfect description of what I have always endeavoured to do.

For as long as I can remember I have been 'in the middle'. I am happy to be a woman, but have always felt limited by it. I enjoy being boyish, but do not want to be a man. I like to be in the middle and reserve the right to be anywhere on the sliding scale that feels right to me at any time. My androgyny and my desire for a 'middle way' is how I define and express myself. I have always been this way and so it was no great decision to begin hormone treatment and to have a bilateral mastectomy to bring out my more boyish aspects. It was as if it created a balance and gave carte blanche for my self-expression.

There are those who might think that the depression and chronic fatigue would be related to a struggle with my gender 'issues', but they are not. I had no struggle with my gender - it just always was. I had no big decision to make. I was very fortunate to have an understanding GP and an opportunity. I would define a transsexual as someone who is unhappy in their existing, gender-specific body, someone feeling trapped and betrayed. I had never felt this. I just felt limited. I did not hate my body; it just appeared to be the wrong vehicle in which to share whatever it was I had to give to the world. I was offered an opportunity to address this and make a change. I knew it was a part of my journey and I pursued it gladly. I always had the full support of my family and friends. I even had the support of the Catholic school where I was teaching at the time, although they were legally obliged to support me under the Sex Discrimination (Gender Reassignment) Regulations 1999 (since replaced by the Equality Act 2010).

Because there is no real social protocol for the 'gender-neutral' and my return to school needed to be 'managed', I gave the school permission to define me in a male role in order to accommodate the changes I was making. My point was that if I genuinely felt neutral, then I did not care what role they assigned to

5

me. And so I explored the extreme of living in a male role for a while, because I could. However, for me it was always about being in the middle, undefined. Limited by my job and position, it was not long before I moved to Manchester, where I could explore my new-found freedom more easily. It was liberating to be part of a much wider and more diverse community. And, whereas I had given away control of my life in unhealthy relationships, exploring my gender and sexuality gave me control over my life again.

My gender treatment has given me the most unique and awe-inspiring understanding of both men and women, of sex and sexuality and of the psychology of gender. I have been given the gift of knowing how a man and a woman thinks, reacts and perceives, a gift that I am able to bring to my work as a therapist. It is also a gift that I bring to my marriage and to all my relationships and interactions.

I was very excited to find out that there is an area of study in META-Health that sheds some light on my gender differences. This area is of course of great interest to me and I continue to study with my Master Trainer, Rob van Overbruggen[3], so that we might share more information about the META-Health view of gender and sexuality. I feel that my personal situation gives me authority to comment on some very specific areas and we will touch on them very briefly in Chapter 7 of this book.

Nothing to lose

I have experienced two very low points in my life. These two 'rock bottoms' both turned out to be fundamental turning points. The first was a depth of depression that gave me the opportunity to explore my gender. I had allowed myself to get into a terrible state over a relationship, desperately hanging on, afraid to let go. I was at the point where the only way was up – or out. 'Out' didn't feel like an option. I didn't want to live, but I didn't particularly want to die either. I think for some people depression is like limbo, where you just want everything to stop. In the depths of my depression I realised that it couldn't

---

3 *Healing Psyche – The Patterns in Psychological Cancer Treatment*, Rob van Overbruggen, PhD, BookSurge Publishing, 2006

get any worse. And if it couldn't get any worse, I had nothing to lose in doing anything I wanted. My thoughts were: 'I have nothing ... I have nothing to lose, so ... I have nothing to lose!' It was like a spiritual realisation. This was the first pivotal point in my life. The second occurred much more recently.

Yet again, I found myself desperate and depressed in a relationship that was my most painful yet. Having promised myself that I would never allow myself to repeat the same mistake, here I was again. Only this time it was worse because I really thought he was 'the one'. What was a 'clean and uncomplicated' relationship when I entered it became a complex and painful love triangle when his ex re-entered the scene. I found myself 'hanging on in there' with the hope of promises, as he rebounded between the two of us for five years. I became more and more ill, depressed, frustrated and angry and used alcohol to cope. I was getting more and more out of control. My frustration at being so impotent in the situation made me become increasingly aggressive. When I drank, I would have violent rages.

Going back to childhood, I remember I had had a fear that I would not be understood - or, more precisely, believed or validated - when I expressed my feelings. My granddad suffered with mental illness and I remember visiting him in the mental hospital one time after he had been sectioned. When I now think back about his behaviour, so much makes sense. I think of his physical and his mental illnesses and understand him better now than I ever thought I would.

When my mum was visiting for Christmas, she tried to help me to overcome my drinking problem. When she remarked that I reminded her of my granddad, I knew something had to change. I knew she was right: I was out of control and needed to do something. This was my second 'rock bottom' and my ultimate turning point. Not only was I was killing myself, but my anger and frustration was dangerous and hurting other people. I was about to lose everything again - most importantly, my sanity.

EFT and Matrix Reimprinting

In the following February, I began searching for help with anger management. Through a series of links I found something called EFT - Emotional Freedom

Techniques[4]. It is a stress-release technique based on Chinese acupuncture and acupressure, in which you tap on specific points along the meridian energy lines that run through the body, in order to move energy and release stress and trapped emotions. This concept of energy and emotion made perfect sense to me as my future husband, Vic, and I had already learned Chinese Health Qigong[5] in China. I completed further training to become an instructor, but on its own it was not enough to bring me out of my depression and my helpless state.

When I stumbled upon EFT, I found that Karl Dawson, EFT Master and creator of the therapy model, Matrix Reimprinting[6], was giving training in Brighton just a mile away. I was compelled to call him immediately. This was not just coincidence; I was ready for this.

I was helpless, a victim of my thoughts and emotions. And, when my emotions got completely overwhelming, I felt no control over my actions. It was as if I was going mad. Drinking and taking drugs numbed my feelings, but also served to give me an excuse for not having control. EFT saved my life.

Karl's course was full, but he took a chance and invited me down to sit in on the second two days of the course - EFT Level 2. I learned EFT and had my first introduction to META-Medicine, which we now call META-Health. My life was transformed over those two days and from that point until I could take the course proper in the following May, I used the EFT meridian tapping technique on everything. All the emotions, the events, the thoughts - everything that kept me in that pit of despair and everything that stirred frustrated, helpless rage inside me. I also learned another energy therapy called EmoTrance - short for Emotional Transformation[7]. Both EFT and EmoTrance have given me a vital relationship with my energy and my emotions, a relationship that I believe we all should have. My emotions are now my guides and I can work

4 See *The EFT Manual*, Gary Craig, Energy Psychology Press, Santa Rosa, CA, 2011
5 See *http://jsqg.sport.org.cn/en/* or *http://www.deyin-taiji.com/what-is-health-qigong*
6 *Matrix Reimprinting Using EFT*, Karl Dawson & Sacha Allenby, Hay House UK Ltd, London, 2010
7 See: *Oceans of Energy - The Patterns & Techniques of EmoTrance, Volume 1*, Silvia Hartmann, PhD, DragonRising, Eastbourne, 2003

with them as e-motions or energy-in-motion. I can process my feelings and return to balance. Balance is the key to health.

Now, no matter what happens in my life, I know I will never go back to where I was. That is just not possible from this new perspective. In recent years, I have enjoyed finding out about myself. Observing my own behaviour has become interesting, rather than scarily out of my control. I see the direct relationship between my emotions and my health and happiness.

> **"If I can share with you just some of what I know so that you can take ownership of your life and your health, I will have done what I set out to do. I offer the gift of freedom. It is yours to take if you are ready."**

I am now a trainer of EFT and EmoTrance, as well as of META-Health. META-Health is the analytical tool to connect the disease in your life, your emotions, your health, with the root-cause events and trauma – however large or small. When you have made those connections, tools such as EFT, EmoTrance and Karl Dawson's Matrix Reimprinting are perfect for releasing the energy from the trauma. Using this pattern of analysis and these applications can bring you a complete shift in understanding and perception and in emotional, psychological and physiological health.

If I can share with you just some of what I know so that you can take ownership of your life and your health, I will have done what I set out to do. I offer the gift of freedom. It is yours to take if you are ready.

What to aim for

META-Health takes the guesswork out of personal development. It brings focus and clarity to your life issues with laser-like precision.

If you are open to the new thinking and discoveries in this book, you will experience a shift in your perspective on life and on health. This can take time to promulgate into daily life. I suspect there may be times when the pace of change will feel a little fast, and at others not fast enough - I know there were such times for me. When I feel that I need to pace myself, I step back and look at the bigger picture. I remind myself of where I was and I reassess where I am now. In turn, this helps me to see where I am aiming for.

> ❝❝ *You will find in-sights and prac-tical tips on how to remind yourself that there is a bigger pic-ture. You will be en-couraged throughout the book to adopt the META perspective. This will enable you to see things from a more re-sourced position, more like the eagle flying above than the worm slinking below.* ❞

To assist you with this, I have tried to offer a way in which you can weave this new and life-changing information into the life in which you currently find yourself. You will find insights and practical tips on how to remind yourself that there is a bigger picture. You will be encouraged throughout the book to adopt the META perspective. This will enable you to see things from a more resourced position, more like the eagle flying above than the worm slinking below.

If you are someone who likes to read a book from cover to cover without putting it down, you may find that I repeat some points quite often. My intention is to allow each chapter to stand alone yet still to hold the full picture of all that is relevant. So, as you go from chapter to chapter, I have reiterated the relevant points as the vista widens. As I build upon the information from previous chapters with the next piece of the puzzle, it's my hope that you will come to embody the overall message of this book. That message is a simple one - you have the power!

From new understandings, small steps can be made. A slight change in trajectory takes you on a new path, to a new future. The new perspectives in this book will either be so different that they will blow your mind, or they will make you breathe a huge sigh of relief when you realise that you were right all along – there IS a better way.

Disclaimer

Although in this book I present a META view of your health situation, is written from my personal perspective and intended simply for complementary health and educational purposes only. Nothing within the book should be taken as advice, or seen as a substitute for the professional advice of a qualified medical practitioner.

I encourage you throughout the book to work with your doctor and health-care providers. If in doubt, always consult a qualified health professional.

1. Are you sick of being sick?

"Health is a state of complete physical, mental and social well-being and not merely the absence of disease or infirmity."

World Health Organization[8]

I t was our first call. I had been speaking with Kevin, my book coach, for almost an hour. He explained how he would coach me through getting my thoughts and ideas out of my head and into some sort of structure, in order to produce this book. It was quite challenging because he forced me to focus and define what I wanted. The more he explained how he worked, the better I felt. I realised I could do it! No sooner had I felt this thought resonate through me than I was hit with a blinding headache.

It made me laugh. I knew exactly why I had the headache, why it had appeared at exactly that time, and even how long it would last.

Illness in our house is now a cause for celebration. So much has our perception of disease changed that on its arrival we are never victims, but curious as to why it is there. My husband will say, 'So what's that about then?' when he has an ache, a pain, a cough or a cold. We will question what has been going on and we will put the pieces together like a jigsaw to find the answer. It is so enlightening to be able to see the connection between what has been going on in the days before and the physical symptoms that manifest as a result. When I was ill in the past, it was a very different story. Trapped in a depression with chronic fatigue and debilitating backache, it seemed endless, with no way out. Even though I had been a Buddhist for years and understood the

---

8 'Preamble to the Constitution of the World Health Organization as adopted by the International Health Conference', New York, 19-22 June, 1946; signed on 22 July 1946 by the representatives of 61 States (Official Records of the World Health Organization, no. 2, p. 100) and entered into force on 7 April 1948.

body-mind connection, it seemed that things were beyond my control. I felt hopeless. The transformation I have undergone since that time is remarkable and, with the knowledge that I have now, I will never go back to that dark place. I will never view illness in the same way again.

Why me? Why now?

Have you ever been ill? Perhaps you're one of those lucky people who have led a relatively healthy life, with only the occasional illness. Most people have had an illness at some time in their life, even if it's just a common cold, but for some illness is a way of life. The problem is that, if you don't understand why something is happening to you, you don't know what options you have to improve matters.

> " As you read through this book I hope that it will become crystal clear that the body is ordered, structured and does not make mistakes. Understanding the specific relationship between stress and dis-ease will help to clarify your health issues and enhance your capability to influence your own healing."

Many people have adopted the belief that the body is a machine that breaks down from time to time. There seem to be so many ways for our bodies to 'go wrong' - diabetes, heart disease, cancer, digestive disorders, dementia, asthma, eczema, fibromyalgia, depression, arthritis, headaches, allergies, to name but a few.

Most of us know someone who is coping with disease – or who has 'dis-ease' in their life, as we prefer to call it. Are you worried about a loved one or is it your job to take care of others? If you are dealing with someone struggling with a mental or physical illness, you will be looking for some way to better understand them and their problems. Not knowing what to do for someone you care for, seeing their pain and anguish and feeling helpless, can lead to stress and illness for the carer too.

So many people are asking the questions: 'Why am I sick?', 'Why this particular illness?', 'Why now?', 'Why me!?' and 'What can I do to heal myself?'

All good questions. Why do some people get sick and others not? Why do I get a bad back and someone else gets bad knees, or a bad neck?

When someone arrives at the office party with a dose of the flu, why do only half the people catch it while the other half don't? And, of the ones who do catch it, why do some get a sore throat, some get sinusitis, some get a chest infection and some get all those symptoms and a fever? Is this simply the random workings of a rampant virus? The answer is 'no'. There is nothing random about it. On the contrary, there is a very specific reason for this differentiation. As you read through this book I hope that it will become crystal clear that the body is ordered, structured and does not make mistakes. Understanding the specific relationship between stress and dis-ease will help to clarify your health issues and enhance your capability to influence your own healing.

Does it run in your family?

What about those who live beneath a cloud of fear that they will develop a pattern of illness inherited from their family line and pass it on to their offspring? Don't the statistics speak for themselves and point to the likelihood of this happening?

Many who were born with an illness, or developed a disease early in life, sadly come to accept the belief that it is not possible to change their inherited state of health and have adapted to the idea of coping with its limitations. From this point of view, the concept of healing is beyond reach and disease seems to be simply an unjust imposition of cruel fate. I recently read a report of a famous actress who chose to have both breasts removed for fear that she might develop the breast cancer that runs in her family[9].

There is big business in genetics, vaccinations and preventative drugs and treatments. Marketing and propaganda can create unnecessary fear in so many of us, even though there is now scientific proof that genes alone do not control our biology. Dr Lipton reveals the new science of epigenetics[10],

9 'My Medical Choice', Angelina Jolie, *New York Times*, 14 May 2013
10 *The Biology of Belief – Unleashing the Power of Consciousness, Matter & Miracles*, Bruce H. Lipton, PhD, Hay House Inc, Carlsbad, CA, USA, 2008

which shows us that our genes are turned on or off by external stimuli. The chemicals in your body are changed by the way your body reacts to your thoughts and perceptions about your environment. These chemical signals are read by your cells and determine which genes are 'switched on' and which are not. This means that genes can be turned on or off depending on the messages they receive; therefore they are not the sole factor in determining our health - the way that you interpret your environment is the determining factor. This new and liberating understanding has yet to filter through the resistance of those that have an investment in maintaining the model of genetic determinism. That model keeps the general public hostage to the idea that we have no control over our bodies or the onset of disease and must seek assistance, usually in the form of drugs, to 'fix' the problem.

META-Health gives a new perspective to see beyond the idea that illness is a mistake or even, as some see it, a punishment.

How do you cope with stress?

What is stress? We tend to perceive stress as a tension or strain in the system - an experience of being overwhelmed in which things are not running smoothly or correctly. There are many types and levels of stress. We have a natural daily rhythm that relies on a certain amount of stress for our daily function and activity, but when we talk about 'stress' we mainly refer to unmanageable thresholds of tension that put a strain on the whole system.

If we consider these thresholds as a balance of energy governing our ability to meet daily demands and stressors, it becomes clearer how diet, environment and, most importantly, emotional resilience play vital roles in our health and wellbeing. All these factors contribute to your general ability to withstand stress and to function under increased demand.

What did you want to do when you grew up? How did you imagine your health and wellbeing? I expect in your youth you didn't pay it much thought. Or, if you are still in your youth and reading this (unless you have a specific illness or health concern), it's probably not something you have dwelt on for too long. By and large, youth is blissfully ignorant of the plethora of illnesses that

> **" " Living in fear or a state of panic that 'everything is out to get us' and that 'the world is a dangerous place' can, in itself, have dire consequences for our health threshold"**

befall the more mature, and yet your ability to manage stress and stressors is hard-wired into you by the age of six years. By the time you turned seven, you had downloaded from your close family and carers all the programmes and codes by which you have interpreted stressful events throughout the rest of your life. The older you get, the harder it is to function if your vital energy has been depleted by stress.

It is our inability to understand *why* an illness occurs that still leaves us in the role of victim. TV, magazines and books often scare us with the threat of this disease or that syndrome. In the extreme, we either ignore the symptoms of disease completely or become hypochondriac. Living in fear or a state of panic that 'everything is out to get us' and that 'the world is a dangerous place' can, in itself, have dire consequences for our health threshold. On the other hand, if we ignore something important for long enough, it doesn't go away, but tends to get worse. Masking the symptoms doesn't solve the problem, but results in a chronic or degenerative illness. This situation can even be further complicated by the side effects of some drugs and allopathic treatments.

Be your own priority

Are you run off your feet most of the time? They say busy people don't have the time to be ill, since they are coping with relationships, family and work commitments. Have you noticed that as soon as you get five minutes to yourself or go on holiday, you get that flu or a stinking cold?

I quite frequently come across people who seem to put their own health and their own needs way down their list of priorities, because they are too busy meeting the needs of others. There is a lot of stress involved in putting other people's needs first, whether it is family, friends or the boss at work. If you are someone carrying a burden of this kind, it is easy to feel unheard and isolated. You can end up assuming that your failing health is just another

17

indicator that you are stuck in a situation not of your own choosing, having to 'get by' rather than being able to flourish in your own life.

Poor health makes it harder to dig yourself out of the hole in which you find yourself. If the world constructed around you does not bring you joy or happiness, the best you may hope for is a few hours of escapism to top up your batteries before you get back on to the treadmill. This scenario is all too common.

Once your threshold of health begins to be compromised, your system has to juggle all the stress that has been accumulating in your life. Drugs may relieve the symptoms, but they may also shift the strain and mask important health messages. If you ignore those signs, you can find yourself on a slippery slope to ill health. With your energy depleted, your immune system is compromised. It takes longer for illnesses to clear and it gets harder to 'bounce back'. When you are in this position, you seem to be constantly fighting ill health and it's a struggle to keep up with even the slightest of stressful situations.

Pain, health and quality of life

Let's look at pain for a moment. Do you have aches and pains? Do they seem to come and go for no apparent reason? Perhaps they seem to be worse in the morning when you first get up or if you sit still for too long. Aches and pains are a part of life - for some, much more than for others. From the odd, passing discomfort to debilitating muscle and joint problems, we accept that it's a common feature of our humanity and that the body is just wearing out. If your illness has led you to a different way of life, you may start to notice a drain on your energy resources and an inability to remain buoyant, even in areas of your life that previously brought you pleasure.

Muscles and joints become weaker and give out under the pressure of daily life. Many come to accept that living in a state of health is not an option for them and instead shift their focus simply to avoiding pain or relieving its symptoms, in order to cope day to day. It has become culturally acceptable to spend a lifetime on painkillers or other medications in order to manage symptoms - we are seldom given alternatives. Most people with chronic pain have forgotten what it was like before they took painkillers and before the pain began. Many people no longer remember what it was like to be healthy. Wouldn't it be great to get that feeling back again?

How then do we measure quality of life? Is it measured by the amount of joy and happiness or the absence of pain and disease?

> *Many people no longer remember what it was like to be healthy. Wouldn't it be great to get that feeling back again?"*

Marking yourself out of 100 per cent, how happy are you? Out of 100 per cent, how healthy are you? How related are these two things for you? Would an improvement in your health bring greater happiness and, vice versa, would a change in your happiness improve your health?

If you could just alleviate one symptom, one illness, or change the fear you have of one disease, how much would that lighten the burden of stressful energy you cope with every day? How much light would that allow back into your life?

Where would you like to be with your own health in a year's time? Although you might have a perfect model of health in mind, it is a good idea to think about this in relation to where you are now, and to how you would like to feel in one year from now. You may just want to maintain your good health and understand your body a little better, so that you can look after it as you grow older. Would you like less physical pain in your life - better breathing maybe? Would you like to be out of the depression you find yourself in? You may even be full of fear because of an illness that seems to have taken you over, or even threatens to take your life. Our illnesses can appear random to the point at which it becomes very difficult to plan or to have any control over our daily lives. From this perspective, we may feel ourselves at the mercy of our bodies - victims of circumstance and the 'bad-health fairy'.

What about my doctor?

Doctors are under a lot of pressure to perform to targets and do their best to cope with increasing patient loads and resulting decreases in time available for each patient. It seems to me to be a highly stressful job. Despite the pressure they are under, some doctors will go the extra mile and, with the help of pamphlets and hand-outs, will offer alternative advice and guidance on stress management and ways to balance emotional wellbeing, alongside their medical care. However, doctors are seldom trained in these areas and so it is extra work, time and effort for which they are not usually recognised or rewarded.

If you are lucky, you may have a doctor who will entertain working along with complementary therapies, giving you more opportunity to address the physical, mental and emotional components of your health in a holistic way, and giving you the best possible chance to return to a healthy, happy life. Sadly, this is not always the case. You could be one of those people who struggle with fear and isolation in the face of your medical diagnosis and prognosis. It is as if your life has been taken out of your hands and everything is happening to you beyond your control. You may feel as though you must 'make the best of it' and 'accept the inevitable'. It can be overwhelming.

Curing symptoms is not the same as healing the causes of ill health and returning to full health. What really empowers people is ownership and responsibility. However, not everyone is ready to let go of ownership and responsibility, and not everyone wants it back.

Whether you're curious or concerned about your own health, or the health of someone you know, you're reading this book because you're open to the possibility that there may be a missing part of the picture. Are you ready to get to know the intelligence of your body, and work with it to take control of your own health and wellbeing?

Is the cost of your health crippling you?

It is one thing to be crippled by illness; it's another to be crippled by the cost of it. Many people feel that they simply cannot afford to be ill, to take time off work because of ill health or, even worse, to have to give up their jobs. Life prospects can change very rapidly once a prognosis of degenerating health has been given. Are you kept awake at night by your fears about being able to look after your family and loved ones with your increasing ill health?

We are lucky in the UK to have the National Health Service. However, did you know that the NHS spends over £8.8 billion on drugs every year?[11] Whose money do you think that is? In the USA, over $300 billion is spent annually on prescription medicines, with almost half the population on a regular prescription regime[12]. Disease is big business.

Just imagine how different things might be if we could invest that money in positive health. What if people could actually get better?

The mind–body connection

Are you curious about how your body works? There is a growing number of people interested in how the body and mind work together. Bookshops dedicate increasingly large sections to 'body-mind-spirit' topics, with a vast array of self-help books from diet and exercise to emotional intelligence and spiritual development. This interest in the body-mind connection is not new; it has been understood for thousands of years and, in more recent times since the seventies, people such as Louise Hay and Deepak Chopra[13] have enlightened us with insights. Louise Hay's book *Heal Your Body*[14] appears on most self-help fanatics' bookshelves, including my own. If you have always been interested in how the body and mind work together, how we get ill, and how we can heal ourselves, this book goes some way to looking at the increasing research in this area and spelling out the connections we have all been searching for.

Most people, including doctors and scientists, have long accepted the connection between stress and illness, yet we still maintain a division when talking about the body-mind-spirit. Since churches took responsibility for the condition of the spirit and science took responsibility for the mechanics of the body, we have struggled to make sense of the interaction between the two. As a result, our thoughts and emotions are seen not as integral, but as abstract and unrelated, to the body. Not all cultures follow this dichotomy. The West

11 *National Statistics 2011-2012*, NHS Information Centre for Health and Social Care
12 'US Drug Costs Dropped in 2012, but Rises Loom', Katie Thomas, *New York Times*, 18 March 2013
13 Deepak Chopra has written more than 70 books, most recently, for example, *Spiritual Solutions – Answers to Life's Greatest Challenges*, Deepak Chopra, Harmony Books, New York, 2012
14 *Heal Your Body – The Mental Causes of Physical Illness and the Metaphysical Way to Overcome Them* (rev. ed.), Louise L. Hay, Hay House Inc., Carlsbad, CA, USA, 2010

now frequently looks to China and India for answers to holistic health as we try to reconnect our body and mind and, in turn, our body-mind and spirit.

In Western medicine, the body is seen as separate and treated as such. If we have a mental disorder, it is also regarded and treated as separate and our emotions are frequently regarded as something to be feared, suppressed or excused.

It is big business these days to 'manage' stress, yet managing the symptoms of stress is not the same as understanding what makes you stressed and unwell in the first place so that you can defuse your triggers.

> *Suppressing our emotions seems to be the number-one Western stress-management tool. If emotions are not processed or released, they will be embodied in illness."*

Although we see a direct correlation between stress and our mental and physical health, we have yet to understand what that connection is. This leaves people isolated in their illnesses, alone with their problems and adrift with their emotions. People are afraid. The more disenfranchised people feel, the more they act from frustration and the more distanced they become from their immediate friends and family as well as from society as a whole. Emotional behaviour is judged to be the cause of the problem, not a symptom, and we move further away from getting to the root of the cultural dis-ease that is surfacing. All because we have turned our backs on the connection between body-mind-spirit and are deaf and blind to the innate language of our emotions.

Have you made a connection between your physical symptoms and your thoughts and feelings? Most people are not even aware what thoughts they do have. Emotions are often regarded as something triggered by other people or external events, so we tend to blame other people and 'manage' our stress responses to avoid people 'getting to us'. Suppressing our emotions seems to be the number-one Western stress-management tool. The danger

22

is that if you suppress your emotions, that energy has to go somewhere else. If emotions are not processed or released, they will be embodied in illness. Then you have the emotions *as well as* the physical or mental illness. Perhaps if you could understand your emotions, you could use them as your internal guidance system, rather than be fearful and suppress them with all the consequences that entails. What we need is a road map that helps us to follow the directions this inner guidance system is giving us. A road map to help us connect the territory of our body to the signs and signposts we are presented with. Maybe then we will not end up lost and running around in circles, but be able to proceed directly to our desired destination and appreciate the journey along the way.

What would it mean for you to be healthy?

If you could wave a magic wand, what would you change about your own health that would improve your quality of life? How different would your life be? Imagine getting up in the morning full of energy, being active and mobile and comfortable in your own body, your aches and pains a thing of the past.

Seduced by the promise of relief, most people use drugs to be rid of their symptoms, only to realise that when they stop using the drugs, the symptoms come back, sometimes more severely. Most people in this situation never manage to break out of the vicious circle of drugs and symptoms. It is possible to bring about an improvement with changes in diet and exercise that certainly can raise one's threshold for coping with illness. Techniques that help you to understand how you think, so that you can stay calmer in the face of stressful events can also play a positive role. But you still have your illness, and you still don't know why you got it. Why you and not someone else? Why at this specific time in your life? And why is this illness getting worse and not getting better? Why won't it go away?

The answer to the questions 'Why me?' and 'Why now?' holds the key to releasing dis-ease from the body. META-Health provides that missing link. If you know why you have an illness, you can prevent it from getting any worse, stop it happening again and know what needs to be done to allow your body to heal. What we also find from understanding the symptoms of dis-ease - the messages from your body - is that the reason for your illness is something very important that you need to know. Acknowledging the thing you need to know can change your view of the world and bring healing on a much deeper level. Not only can you have an impact on your own health, but you can also change your life and have more freedom and more joy.

This book contains an answer to all these problems. In understanding the fuller picture and the purpose of the changes that your body has made, you will understand what caused those changes. If, like me, you are looking for answers and are ready to learn what you can do to take back your health I promise you this book could change your life.

2. META-Health - the missing link

"Meta (from the Greek preposition μετά = "after", "beyond", "adjacent", "self") ... In epistemology, the prefix meta- is used to mean about (its own category). For example, metadata are also data about data." **Wikipedia**

Imagine that the body you have right at this moment, in the condition that it is in right now, is your greatest gift. Hard to imagine?

There are messages locked inside your body. If you ignore them, or cannot read them, they are expressed in the symptoms of dis-ease.

Do you have pain, dis-ease, infection? What if you understood the reason for your specific ailment? What if you understood the infection you had, or knew exactly *why* your right ankle and knee was hurting, or why you had a stomach ulcer? Do you think that such information might allow you to support your body in its return to health?

Maybe it's time to re-examine your symptoms and bring in a new perspective - one that allows you to re-associate with the root cause of your dis-ease. If you learned to pay more attention to your specific symptoms, because you knew that there was a message in them for you, and if you could read the signs of your symptoms, you might be surprised by what they reveal. If you really acknowledged that your body is trying to tell you something, maybe you would listen a little harder.

If you are going to unravel the mysteries of your illness, you need to know the specific questions to ask to lead you back to the root cause. You will need to

25

We humans, unlike animals in the wild, do not release our shocks and traumas so easily. Instead, we tend to re-live unresolved situations in a continued attempt to resolve them. "

understand the unique and ordered way in which the body is created and why, in its divine intelligence, the body does not make a mistake.

Open your mind to the possibility that, if you have not been able to deal with a trauma or event on a mental or emotional level, your body will adapt to compensate. Once you understand the underlying reason for the change that occurs in your body, you can uncover the traumatic event that triggered it and so come to understand the message that your body is giving you. These natural bio-logical responses can be observed in animals and humans alike and are part of our fundamental development and evolution.

Our bodily responses to stimuli are animalistic insofar as we respond physically in the same way that an animal in the wild would respond. If we fear the boss's anger, for example, our hearts might begin to race, just as that of a deer preparing to flee the wrath of a marauding wolf. However, we humans have evolved into complex, social animals whose natural responses are inhibited by a web of social rules and regulations. While our underlying animalistic stimulus perceives a threat, we lack the freedom to respond as we might in the wild. We cannot fight neither can we flee, so we experience a 'freeze' response. This can leave us caught in the process of an over-stimulated bodily response without the necessary release, thus creating an illness.

We humans, unlike animals in the wild, do not release our shocks and traumas so easily. Instead, we tend to re-live unresolved situations in a continued attempt to resolve them. We fixate upon and go over our past experiences and we worry and fret about the future. This is because information from a traumatic event stays trapped, frozen in our energy and awaiting an opportunity for resolution. This accumulation of small and large traumas stored in the system is exhibited as stress. To compensate, the body continues to adapt in an attempt to assist us to protect ourselves against the ongoing and unresolved threat, until the danger has passed and the issue is resolved. Then the body will enter into repair.

An awareness of the specific changes your body makes can give you new insight into what is going on in your life to cause the reactions. Making these connections gives you the power to make changes in your life, enabling you to support your innate power to heal.

Discovering the connection

The key principles of META-Health embody the discoveries of Dr Ryke Geerd Hamer[15], the founder of 'Germanic New Medicine®', but take them further into a new healing paradigm.

In 1978 Dr Hamer, a German GP and specialist in internal medicine, experienced a tragic event. He received a call late one night, to be told that his only son, Dirk, had been accidentally shot. Three months later Dirk died, leaving Dr Hamer devastated. A short time after this shock, Dr Hamer developed testicular cancer. As he'd been healthy all his life, he suspected that there could be a connection between his crippling loss and the onset of his cancer. While working in a German university clinic Dr Hamer began to research this theory, interviewing every woman patient who had had ovarian cysts. He found that every one of the women, without exception, had experienced the shock of losing a loved one prior to the onset of their disease. Over the next twenty years, Dr Hamer went on to do extensive research and made further discoveries, backed by empirical evidence from tens of thousands of cases. On the basis of this evidence, he was able to develop a new framework of findings and principles later called the 'Germanic New Medicine®'. However, Hamer faced great hostility from the established medical profession. The nature of his findings was a challenge to convention and Dr Hamer's strong views about the intervention of medicine in the natural biological process of disease, has caused much controversy.

---

15 'Germanic New Medicine® - The Five Biological Laws of the New Medicine', presentation by Dr Ryke Geerd Hamer to the *First International Congress on Complementary and Alternative Medical Cancer Treatment*, Madrid, May 2005

Just as Isaac Newton observed the universal law of gravity in action and was able to define it and give it tangible and measurable qualities to prove its existence, so too Hamer observed and defined certain natural, biological processes related to the dis-ease process.

> ❝ *Change is frightening for people. But the need for change is vital. Nothing stays the same and resistance to change can even cause dis-ease.* ❞

Newton did not 'invent' gravity. He had a realisation. He was able to test and prove his theory, resulting in it becoming the most widely accepted theory of gravitational pull today. Indeed, this theory is now so much part of our culture that we do not even notice or question it. For example, did you think the last time that you stepped on the weighing scales that your weight was being calculated by measuring the gravitational pull on the mass of your body? There seems to be a natural logic, a truth, to Newton's theories that fits our way of thinking and, until such time as another insight takes us further, we adopt it as the most logical. New insights and theories are challenging and may be resisted with great effort until it becomes too unsatisfactory to stick with the old theories that no longer serve us. We will reject new insights and, even if it's so obvious that we are staring the answer in the face, we will look the other way rather than acknowledge the need for us to change our view. Change is frightening for people. But the need for change is vital. Nothing stays the same and resistance to change can even cause dis-ease. For some, change will only happen when the pain of staying the same is greater than the pain of changing.

However, as our technological capabilities increase we are able to test and measure forces and theories in a way that was not possible before. This has led to a more scientific understanding of unseen forces such as gravity, magnetism, electricity, radio waves, and the human energy field. What was once condemned as witchcraft is now hailed as science. Now, through the work of scientists such as Dr Bruce Lipton[16], Dr Rupert Sheldrake[17] and Dr David Hamilton[18], we are coming full circle to understanding the body-mind connection in a scientific light. Whereas spirituality had previously been divorced from science as being the monopoly of religion, it is now becoming reunited with science to make the picture whole once again.

Those with a vested interest in keeping things the way they are will always resist new information to protect their control and monopoly. But the truth is evidential. The more people are open to the truth and are able to see the evidence in their own lives, the more it will become acceptable to be open to new information and evidence.

Although Dr Hamer did not discover anything new in terms of evolution, he brought to our attention the way things work together in such a committed and scrupulously scientific way that we are deeply indebted to him. His observations can be tested, verified and seen in action in everyday life. Knowing this information gives us a choice. However, we have to make a clear distinction here between knowledge of how things work in the body and choosing how that information should be used. The emphasis is very much on awareness and responsibility. Each individual is responsible for making their own choices and ultimately for assisting in their own healing.

Inspired by Dr Hamer's work, Johannes R. Fisslinger[19] and Dr Anton Bader, another German GP, founded the International META-Medicine Association (IMMA) in 2004. The Association bases its work upon the model that Hamer had developed to show the conflict-organ connection, but has gradually expanded this understanding in many important ways. IMMA maintains a

---

16 *The Biology of Belief - Unleashing the Power of Consciousness, Matter & Miracles*, Bruce H. Lipton PhD, op. cit.
17 *Morphic Resonance - The Nature of Formative Causation*, Rupert Sheldrake PhD, Park Street Press, Vermont, 1981
18 It's the Thought that Counts - Why Mind over Matter Really Works, David R. Hamilton PhD, Hay House UK Ltd, London, 2005
19 *META-Health, De-Coding Your Body's Intelligence*, Johannes R. Fisslinger, META-Health Publishing, Marina Del Rey, CA, 2013.
See also *www.metahealthuniversity.com*

completely integrative approach to health and takes great care to work with health professionals from all disciplines.

The principles of META-Health

The International META-Medicine Association comprises medical doctors and health professionals from all over the world and, while acknowledging Dr Hamer's immense contribution, has developed a far wider-reaching model of health and healing that integrates the biological, psychological and social aspects of health into a new paradigm. In this approach, modern medical practice as well as alternative and complementary therapies are combined with the individual's own innate ability to heal her/himself. The aim of META-Health professionals is to empower individuals with the confidence to take ownership of their health by identifying the root causes of illness and disease. What begins as a purely biological analysis of cellular changes may become a very deep, emotional and even spiritual message.

> " *The aim of META-Health professionals is to empower individuals with the confidence to take ownership of their health by identifying the root causes of illness and disease.* "

The ten principles that underlie the META-Health paradigm are as follows:

1. There is an **ORDER** and structure to the development and evolution of the brain and organ tissue.
2. There is an order and **STRUCTURE** to the communication between the organ-brain-psyche.
3. The starting point of dis-ease is a **TRAUMATIC** life experience.
4. Dis-ease is a **PROCESS** which takes place in two determinable phases.
5. Fungi, microbes, bacteria and viruses are bio-logical **HELPERS**.
6. Every symptom has a bio-logical and psychological **MEANING**.
7. **AWARENESS** of this connection is a prerequisite for personal growth and health.
8. There is a body-mind-spirit and social **CONNECTION**.
9. The individual is **RESPONSIBLE** for acquiring knowledge and for making her/his own decisions in regard to her/his own wellbeing.
10. **SELF-HEALING** is integrative with all therapies and treatments.

Use the information in the following pages to find these connections for yourself in your own life, go on a journey of enquiry and discovery, and be curious about your own capabilities and power. I am excited to share this information with you. Hopefully, it will enable you to adopt a new perspective on your health and your life. What you do with that new vista of possibilities is for you to decide. As a META-Health professional, I can help you to make connections between your body and the events in your life or thoughts that may be undermining your health. It is not my place to advise you on your medical condition or on what medical advice to take. Rather, it is my aim to empower you with the information to make informed choices for yourself. I strongly encourage you to work with your doctor or therapist on the issues that arise, in order to create the best path to a fuller recovery and long-term health. Take the initiative to do all that you can for yourself.

This META understanding profoundly changes the way in which we work with health and healing. Rather than focus on disease and fighting or managing the symptoms of disease, these principles give us the framework to focus on creating and maintaining health. They help us to analyse exactly what is needed on all levels to bring the body through its natural healing processes.

Law and order

In order to make sense of what the body is doing on a survival level, we need to revisit some basic biology. Understanding the order and structure of the body gives us our first pieces of the puzzle.

You are a highly intelligent and ordered being. There are no mistakes in nature and each part of you - from your quarks and atoms to your cells and organs - is organised and structured with a unique and specific function and purpose. This structure and order supports a natural logic that enables your body and mind to function as one. It is now possible to see this structure in the connection between organ, brain and psyche.

The development of an organism from its origins is called ontogenesis or ontogeny. The study of this process, like other areas we will examine, is a scientific discipline already established independently of META-Health. We'll examine some of this area in enough detail to clarify the organ-brain-psyche connection. Research for yourself the amazing discoveries in neurology, embryology, epigenetics, pathology, anatomy and physiology. You will find some very interesting information that will further consolidate your understanding of how intelligent and organised your body really is.

Once you understand how the findings from these different disciplines are interconnected, you will be able to decode the body's intelligence and interpret the META messages from your body. By better understanding the relationships between the different functions of the brain and the body, you can begin to map the way in which they work together when stimulated by a shock or conflict, or by a trigger event that takes you back to such a shock.

How the brain is ordered

There is a pattern and order to the structure of the brain. The brain has different 'departments' that control the functions of different parts of the body. The brain has been studied and mapped in great detail by doctors and scientists over the years to show how every part of the body has a corresponding connection to the brain. The brain evolved in stages as humans evolved. These stages are characterised by four distinct brain layers. The older inner brain layers are responsible for basic survival functions and the new outer brain layers govern our social interactions with the world about us. We have four main brain layers:

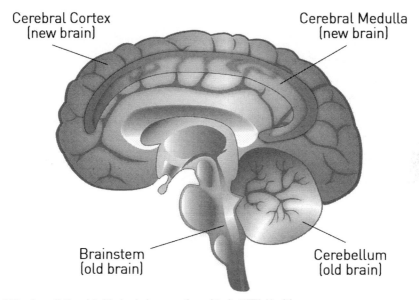

Cerebral Cortex
(new brain)

Cerebral Medulla
(new brain)

Brainstem
(old brain)

Cerebellum
(old brain)

Fig.2 The four distinguishable brain layers referred to in META-Health

- Brainstem (old brain)
- Cerebellum (old brain)
- Cerebral medulla (new brain)
- Cerebral cortex (new brain)

33

The medical term 'medulla' means the inner region of an organ, for example the renal medulla is the innermost part of the kidney. When we refer to the cerebral medulla, we mean the inner region of the cerebrum, sometimes referred to as 'white matter'. We refer to the 'grey matter' of the cerebrum as the cerebral cortex.

How the body tissue is ordered

At day sixteen in the development of an embryo in the womb, the cell structure begins to separate into three different types of 'germ layer'. They are called germ layers in the sense that they are the 'germ' of a cell - the beginning, like the germ of an idea. There are three such germ layers and all cells in the human body are made from one or another type of these three germ layers.

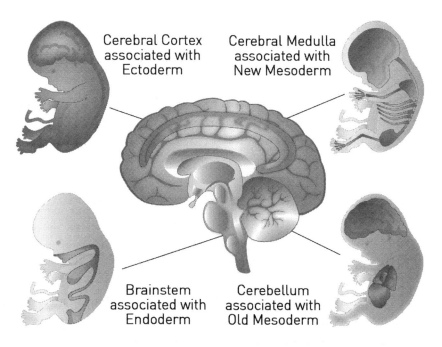

Cerebral Cortex associated with Ectoderm

Cerebral Medulla associated with New Mesoderm

Brainstem associated with Endoderm

Cerebellum associated with Old Mesoderm

Fig.3 The four brain layers and their associated germ layers

The three germ layers are:

- Endoderm (inner germ layer)
- Mesoderm (middle germ layer)
- Ectoderm (outer germ layer).

The connection between brain and body

The four brain layers derive from the three germ layers in an ordered way and operate together to complete a specific theme and function:

- Brainstem (endoderm)
- Cerebellum (old mesoderm)
- Cerebral medulla (new mesoderm)
- Cerebral cortex (ectoderm).

All the organs of the body are constructed from cells derived from one of these three germ layers and sometimes from a combination of these, depending on how complex are their functions and purposes.

Evolution and development

Because we understand the connection between the brain layers and the germ layers and the way that human beings evolved over time, it is possible to identify 'themes' governing the functions of the four brain layers and how they relate to corresponding organ tissues.

These themes relate closely to the periods of our development from simple creatures emerging from the primeval swamp to the complex social beings that we are today. Broadly defined, they are as follows:

- **Brainstem** - Theme: Digestion and survival of the species, including reproduction and breathing.

35

The most basic level of animal survival.

This brain layer corresponds with the tissues made from endoderm germ cells, including the tissue of the tonsils, pituitary gland, liver parenchyma, thyroid gland, middle ear, tear ducts, intestine, uterus, ovaries, testicles, bladder, colon, rectum, prostate and lung alveoli among others.

- **Cerebellum** – Theme: Protection and integrity, also including issues related to feeling ugly.
  The crude beginnings of interaction with the surrounding environment.

  This brain layer corresponds with tissues made from earlier-developed mesoderm germ cells such as that in the dermis of the skin, the meninges, the pericardium, the peritoneum and the pleura.

- **Cerebral medulla** – Theme: Movement and strength, needing to be good enough or strong enough to do something.
  The phase of exploration and activity in the world.

  This brain layer corresponds with tissues formed from later-developed mesoderm germ cells such as that in tendons, ligaments, joints, muscles and bones, connective tissue, tooth bone, the adrenal cortex, blood vessels, arteries, veins, and the lymph glands among others.

- **Cerebral cortex** – Theme: Social, territorial and contact.
  The stage of social interaction with our fellow beings in groups.
  This brain layer corresponds to tissue formed from ectoderm germ cells; it includes tissues of the tongue, nose, bronchi, small curvature of the stomach, vagina, coronary arteries and veins, thalamus, and skin epidermis among others.

The bio-logical purpose

Every tissue in the body reacts in a manner specific to its function and in accordance with its associated brain layer and theme. When we know this, we can begin to understand what bio-logical reason is at work when there is a change in cell activity.

At our current stage of evolution, we have evolved beyond the primal animal into conscious beings and are able to interpret situations in both a literal and a metaphorical way. A direct physical attack is literally a life-threatening event. However, as we have developed into highly conscious, social beings, we may also experience an attack to the psychological 'self' or interpret a metaphorical event as a real attack.

> *Every tissue in the body reacts in a manner specific to its function and in accordance with its associated brain layer and theme. When we know this, we can begin to understand what bio-logical reason is at work when there is a change in cell activity.*

Cellular changes that take place in the body are a fundamental adjustment to a threat or stressor. It could be a real, direct threat, such as someone attempting to stab me in the heart. However, equally, if I feel that someone metaphorically stabbed me in the heart, I will have the same biological response. In both these cases, the pericardium, the protective sack around the heart, will thicken to protect the heart.

Once you have ruled out the possibility of a literal attack or life-threatening situation, it is possible to explore the metaphor that the body has translated and to which it has provided a physiological response. This is not the same as imagining an illness - this is still a very real, bio-logical response to the perception of a real threat to survival.

This goes some way to understanding tissue reactions. However, we need much more information in order to pinpoint specific event, trigger or thought that caused the response and, in cases such as chronic disease, that continues to hold the illness in place.

The brain receives the instruction

When a person experiences a traumatic experience (referred to in META-Health as a 'conflict-shock'), the information is received in a specific area of the brain. As Dr Robert Scaer[20], a leading expert in trauma, says: 'All it takes for a trauma to occur is a state of helplessness and a threat to survival.' In META-Health we also refer to the conflict-shock as a 'UDIN', because it is:

> **U**nexpected,
> **D**ramatic,
> **I**solating, leaving the individual with
> **N**o strategy to deal with it.

In the past, this UDIN has also been referred to as a Significant Emotional Event, or SEE. Personally, I prefer this term as it reflects the subjectivity of the client's perception.

When a trauma that meets these criteria is perceived, the information is received in a specific area of the brain, which we call a relay. This is the part of the brain that corresponds to the relevant organ required to respond to that specific traumatic experience. For example, when perceiving that you are unable to prevent someone from entering or leaving your territory, an impulse will be received in the front right part of the cortex, which is associated with the tissue of bronchial mucous membranes (mucosa[21]). This organ-brain-psyche reaction happens simultaneously at the moment of the trauma. Most remarkably, the impact point of this information received in the brain is visible on a Computer Tomography (CT, formerly called Computer Axial Tomography or CAT) scan.

---

20 *The Body Bears the Burden – Trauma, Dissociation and Disease* (2nd ed.), Robert C. Scaer MD, Routledge, New York, 2007
21 Mucosa: linings of mostly endodermal origin, covered in epithelium, which are involved in absorption and secretion. They line cavities that are exposed to the external environment and internal organs. They are at several places contiguous with skin: at the nostrils, the lips of the mouth, the eyelids, the ears, the genital area, and the anus. (Wikipedia)

Since the early 1970s, CT scans have been an important tool in medical diagnosis. Specialist equipment produces computer-processed X-rays of the body, a slice at a time. These CT scans are used to show up irregularities and abnormalities inside the body. Dr Hamer noticed that on the brain CT scans of his patients there were distinct, irregular markings in specific locations on the brain. These markings were always in the position in the brain that corresponded to whatever organ would be engaged in responding to the trauma that the patient had suffered.

After extensive study into the CT scans of many thousands of patients, it has been possible to map the impact points of different types of shock-conflict in specific areas of the brain across the four different brain layers. These brain charts form a fundamental tool in META-Health root-cause analysis and allow us to verify the connection between the type of trauma and the brain's and organ's response to it.

Clear marking on CT
scan of active conflict in
Brainstem area associated with
Right Kidney Collecting Tubules

META-Health map of
Brainstem with conflict
areas defined for use
in META-Health analysis

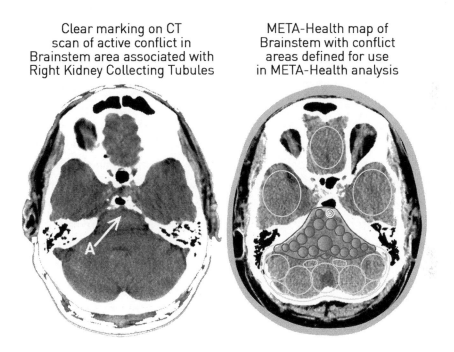

Fig.4 Example CT brain scan with corresponding META-Health chart

39

Now that the impact points have been mapped across many case studies, it is no longer necessary to take a CT scan each time we do an analysis. Instead, we can use our knowledge of the mapped information to work our way via the symptoms of the organ-tissue response back to the shock-conflict that caused it. However, if a patient or client does have a CT scan from a previous test, it is possible for an expert to analyse purely from the scan the exact organ response and the original conflict-shock from which it derives. A specialist trained in the reading of a CT scan can also tell the state of the conflict (whether it is active and still running or has been resolved) and can even tell the approximate age of the client at the time of the trauma. I must admit this is not something I do myself. I use the information that has been mapped and, with subtle questioning techniques, formulate a timeline of symptoms, relevant triggers and patterns so that, together with the client and their doctor, I can build a clear picture of the dis-ease, its origins and any contributing factors.

When you map this information, your symptoms begin to become signposts, so that what was once a confusing, random illness becomes a clear and bio-logical response. This is always the first step to healing – knowing the real reason behind your illness.

Your body always does as it's told

Faced with a trauma, the body-mind reacts simultaneously. The information is received in the brain at a very specific impact point that remains visible on a CT scan. As I mentioned before, this is the case if you experience a real, life-threatening trauma such as, for example, an attack to the head, or equally if you simply perceive a threat that is not actually happening in the present. We may have experienced a past event that we continue to re-live, or we may fear that a situation could occur based on a series of other perceptions. The body does not know the difference between a real and a perceived threat. The impact on the brain relay and the message to the organ is the same. If I have a traumatic experience that feels like a metaphoric attack to the head, such as someone attacking my intellect, this trauma will affect my reaction in the same manner as if it were readying itself for a real blow to the skull. In both the 'real' trauma and the 'perceived' trauma, the information

40

would impact a relay in the cerebellum and would trigger a thickening of the membrane (meninges) between the brain and the skull, in order to cushion the brain from an impending impact.

Let us examine an example for each brain layer:

- **Brainstem** – Theme: Digestion and survival; reproduction.
  Issue: prostate cancer. Biological reason: need to produce more ejaculate to spread more seed.

  Example: *Alan's prostate problems began not long after his wife had left him for a younger man and he felt that his manhood had been undermined.*

- **Cerebellum** - Theme: Protection and integrity.
  Issue: facial acne. Biological reason: feeling ugly or a need to protect (be thicker-skinned) in that area.

  Example: *during her teenage years, Sarah suddenly developed a bad case of acne on her face. She admitted to feeling rather shy and aware of the opposite sex and to feeling very conscious about her looks and what people thought of her.*

- **Cerebral medulla** – Theme: Movement and strength.
  Issue: painful and stiff neck. Biological reason: need to be stronger in this area, to hold my head high.

  Example: *David complained of persistent neck pain. In the course of discussion, he pointed out that although he had good qualifications, he was constantly overlooked for promotion in his job and felt himself to be the target of an injustice against which he could do nothing.*

- **Cerebral cortex** - Theme: Social, territorial and contact. Issue: blocked nose and sinuses. Biological reason: need to get fresher, clearer or more air into the senses.

  Example: *June presented with persistently blocked and aching sinuses. During analysis she admitted that she was constantly annoyed by the behaviour of her partner; she wanted him to change his ways and expressed her view that the current situation 'stank'.*

We are modern-day animals

As social animals we are obliged to respond in a 'civilised' manner. Although our triggers may prompt our bodies to react in a natural, animalistic way, it is not possible for us to give full rein to our basic instincts in the way that an animal could. I know this seems obvious: I am sure that you would not consciously dream of urinating around your space at work to mark out your territory, just as you wouldn't bite someone if you felt verbally attacked! Social protocol dictates that we do not act like animals. We are more highly evolved; we are conscious beings and have choice.

> **"** *I am sure that you would not consciously dream of urinating around your space at work to mark out your territory, just as you wouldn't bite someone if you felt verbally attacked! Social protocol dictates that we do not act like animals.* **"**

It would seem that we are, on the one hand, highly evolved and yet, on a subconscious level, the body still reacts in a basic, animalistic way. The body does exactly what it is instructed or triggered to do. You might think then that disease is a mistake and that the body is making that mistake by responding in such a way, but is that really what is happening? The body will only do what it is told to do. It will respond dutifully and lovingly to the messages it is sent and do all in its power to adjust, change and to compensate for the problems that you experience in the world around you. Your body will accommodate to the world as you perceive it.

Cause and effect

I hope you have begun to see how amazing nature is and how ordered and intelligent your body is. Each of us is a collection of some 50 trillion cells. Every cell has a specific function and purpose. When stimulated to do so, our body can increase or decrease the cells that perform a specific function to bring about a change in the body to cope with greater stress on that area. The cells can be sent the message to adjust to stress and to enter into repair and regeneration. We have an innate ability to heal ourselves.

Our 50 trillion cells are made up of proteins. There are over 100,000 proteins in every cell. There are three things that may interfere with the healthy functioning of a protein, that is, cause dis-ease. They are:

- **A direct, physical trauma** A blow to the head, for example, would interfere with the signals to the proteins.
- **A chemical or toxin** that interferes with the signals to the proteins.
- **An energetic signal** A thought that sends an incorrect message to a cell. If we realise that electro-magnetic energy is 100 times more effective at transmitting information than chemicals, we may be able to understand how the body can react so immediately to threats or perceived threats. We might also start to see why our thoughts are far more powerful than most medications. Why is it, for example, that in trial after trial patients who are unknowingly given sugar pills that have no chemical effect frequently improve at rates equal to, and even in excess of, those who are given expensive prescription drugs? This so-called 'placebo effect' demonstrates very well that what we believe dictates how our bodies will react.

If a person is in an environment that poses a direct threat - a war zone or an abusive relationship, for example - the perception of danger is very real and so the message of danger to the body is real. It would be detrimental to stay in any situation like this for a long time, but the body's adjustments to cope with the extra stress on the system would help survival over a short period. These signals serve a correct purpose and could be life-saving. However, if the person continues to fear the same dangers once the dangerous situation is past, if she/he re-lives those events and continues to send the same signals to the body, the body will continue to react in the same way. It will release the same chemicals and stimulate the same changes to the cell tissue. To the body, there is no difference between the actual event and the memory of it. For optimal health, it becomes imperative to create the correct environment for healthy cells and healthy cell function. Conversely, if the body is in poor health, we can see that there is either a direct threat or that incorrect messages are being transmitted to the body and causing dis-ease.

Prevention is better than cure

It is because we have not been listening to our emotions and our bodies that we have got into a mess. We have symptoms that make no sense to us, illnesses that appear to be a betrayal of all that we aspire to. Our energetic systems are storing information that we need to process so that we can be healthy and robust and our bodies can be healed. Other cultures, such as the Chinese and Indian through traditional Chinese medicine and Ayurvedic medicine, continue to recognise the integral connection between our thoughts and emotions and our organs. Traditionally, Chinese medicine is a preventative practice. In ancient China, doctors were paid while they maintained their clients' good health, but payment ceased all the while they were sick!

The truth of the matter is that dis-ease happens. It happens to everyone, but the degree to which it happens and the effect it has is dependent on the basic wellbeing of the individual. A swift recovery, which for some can even mean a lack of symptoms, depends on mental and physical health and, above all, emotional health. Much as people try to avoid or deny the relevance of emotions, they form our guidance system.

Emotional guidance

We are hard-wired to be different as men and women. Traditionally men are hunters while women tend the nest. Our skills have developed differently so that we may perform these basic roles and, even in a society of equal roles and opportunities, this remains true on a purely biological level.

Even in primitive times, both men and women relied on intuition and emotion to perform these basic functions. Being nearer to our animal origins, both genders were more in touch with intuition and emotions. We listened to our gut feelings, we tuned into our senses and trusted when something felt dangerous, or we felt moved to respond. We took feedback from our heart, mind and body and acted naturally upon the information. However, in our vastly more complex societies, we have since learned to ignore our own intuitions and to follow the instructions and guidance of others. We are taught to adopt hand-me-down beliefs and are 'sold' answers to our problems. We no longer function as holistic beings. We look outside ourselves for cures.

This real sensation in your body is your emotional energy. It is your guidance mechanism and is working and talking to you all the time. By allowing your emotions to come through and by listening to what they have to say, you can process the energy so that it does not get embodied as dis-ease. If you reconnect with your body as an integral part of your energetic being, including your emotions, you will be able to achieve health and balance. You can become whole again.

This chapter has given an overview of the relationship between our thoughts and the way in which they are received and processed by our brains and our organs. Now we need to understand how this occurs as a process. These changes in the body are not static and happen as part of a clearly definable process.

3. Your body doesn't make mistakes

Gratitude unlocks the fullness of life. It turns what we have into enough, and more. It turns denial into acceptance, chaos into order, confusion into clarity. It can turn a meal into a feast, a house into a home, a stranger into a friend."

Melody Beattie[22]

Just think what a loving and supportive relationship you could have with your body if you knew for certain that it was constantly working to support and protect you. You could be best friends, loving, kind and encouraging.

This relationship could start right now, even if you do not understand exactly what your body is doing on your behalf at the moment. You might not like what is happening in your body, but you are, in fact, getting the results now of exactly what your body has been 'told' to do to help you, based on your past experiences.

'META' in this context means 'in a position above and beyond something'. We will also explore how it explains exactly what the body is doing when faced with a trauma or event to which it needs to respond. In this sense, 'META' stands for:

M – Meaningful
E – Emotional
T – Tissue
A – Adaptation

22 *Co-Dependent No More – How to Stop Controlling Others and Start Caring for Yourself* (2nd ed.), Melody Beattie, Hazelden Foundation, Center City, USA, 1992

M - Meaningful

Your body is an elegantly designed and structured organism. The four brain layers - the brainstem, the cerebellum, the cerebral medulla and the cerebral cortex - have evolved to correspond with specific organs and tissues. These organs and tissues have specific functions. As a supremely ordered organism, the human body does not make mistakes in its functioning. There is meaning in every response, even if we don't immediately understand what it is. Once you do understand what the function of a change is, you may understand what stimulus or trigger began that change.

The Trigger

What is a trigger? Once a traumatic event has happened and you have learned that a certain set of circumstances may spell danger or cause you pain, a trigger is anything that reminds you of the original event.

You may be aware of an initial, traumatic life event, but often we are not aware what our triggers are. We are only aware of how we feel when we have been triggered. This is because at the time of a trauma the subconscious mind will take a snapshot of everything in our surroundings (all sights, smells, sounds and energies) and it will also identify and record everything that is present in our internal system at the time (all foods, chemicals, etc). The subconscious mind now has a record of potential dangers that it wishes to avoid in future, because they may cause the same reaction as the original trauma. So, when the subconscious encounters a situation that bears similarities to our original traumatic event, it 'triggers' or sets off a warning or protective response in the body. Very often, however, you may not be aware what the connection is between the reaction that you have now and the original traumatic event - it might be any one of the elements captured by the subconscious snapshot. This is also the mechanism through which we develop allergies and intolerances.

For example, a woman with an extremely severe allergy to coffee, including its sight and smell, was, with professional help, able to trace her reaction back to the many cups of coffee she had consumed in the home for battered women where she had taken refuge after being beaten up by her husband. As she and her fellow residents sat in the kitchen talking about their traumas, the coffee had become associated in her unconscious mind with those highly traumatic stories and so triggered an array of symptoms associated with the original traumas.

> **What is a trigger? Once a traumatic event has happened and you have learned that a certain set of circumstances may spell danger or cause you pain, a trigger is anything that reminds you of the original event."**

Once you have been triggered, it is difficult to be aware of what has caused you to feel the effects, because the trigger will bypass your conscious awareness to be directly processed by the subconscious mind. On the surface, you won't understand what changed, but when it happens you may experience disturbances in your mood or in your health. Because it has all happened subconsciously, you are not consciously aware of the connections. So you assume that the way people make you feel, or the way that things 'happen to you' is someone else's fault or 'just the way things are'; often, you make no correlation between the everyday experiences that you face and the symptoms present in your body. You don't initially recognise the trigger that created your symptoms, just as the lady with the coffee allergy had not made the connection between coffee and her original trauma.

Just think for a moment. Can you recall an upsetting event or situation, or perhaps something that is upsetting you at the moment? Is there something that you find yourself running over in your head, a thought you are unable to let go of? Perhaps something happened and you find that you are still going over what was said and done, or what should have been said or done? Your mind is trying to resolve the issue so that you can let it go, but it still bugs you and you still have some emotional charge around it. This is typically recognised as experiencing some level of stress.

49

When stressed, you will search for a way to resolve the issue and your mind will try to figure out what to do, while your body compensates in order to cope with the increased stress. Here are some perceptions and reactions that you might experience in an everyday situation:

- You were so angry and could not understand why someone would behave in such a way.
- You thought that someone thought you were a bad person and might tell everyone else and you would lose face.
- You wanted to stand up for yourself to someone in authority, but were not able to do so.
- You felt that people did not take you seriously because you were unable to define your position and make your views clear.

None of these situations is necessarily drastic, but what is a small and passing concern for one person can be overpowering and all-consuming for another.

Short bio-logical programmes

On a bio-logical level, all these triggered reactions will be swiftly handled by a brief adaptation of your bodily responses, in keeping with their purposes and functions, to maintain your emotional equilibrium while you deal with daily occurrences. These brief reactions often pass unnoticed. It is only when we are unable to escape the danger, or intellectually or emotionally to let go of situations, that we enter into a dis-ease process.

If we associate the examples listed above with the bio-logical need that the person experienced at the time in order to do things better in future, we will understand more clearly why the body reacts the way it does:

- **Emotional event** - You were so angry and could not understand why someone would behave in such a way.

Required resolution - You need to be able to work out and digest someone's behaviour.

Bio-logical tissue adaptation - Extra cells are created in the small or large intestine, so that the incomprehensible behaviour that is being held onto can be broken down, digested and absorbed.

Typical dis-ease - IBS (irritable bowel syndrome) with alternating constipation and diarrhoea and, in very severe cases, bowel cancer.

- **Emotional event** - You believed that someone thought you were a bad person and might tell everyone else and you would lose face.

  Required resolution - You need to be thicker-skinned next time you face these people, in case they think badly of you.

  Bio-logical tissue adaptation - A thickening of the dermis layer of skin, which protects us from how others perceive us.

  Typical dis-ease - Noticed as red and painful, swelling acne under the skin, followed by an outbreak of acne.

- **Emotional event** - You wanted to stand up for yourself to someone in authority, but were not able to do so.

  Required resolution - You need to be stronger and able to stand tall when facing up to the authority figure.

  Bio-logical tissue adaptation - A weakness followed by a strengthening of the muscles and bones in the thoracic area of the spine (just as a bodybuilder would damage a muscle on purpose with specific weight-lifting exercises, to allow it to heal stronger).

Typical dis-ease - If there is ongoing stress, a weakening of the thoracic spine, causing round shoulders.

- **Emotional event** - You felt that people did not take you seriously because you were unable to define your position and make your views clear.

  Required resolution - You need to be decisive and make a bold statement of your position so that your position is understood.

  Bio-logical tissue adaptation - In animals, the most definite and bold way to make a statement is to defecate on the spot. Biologically a human will experience a decrease in cells of the rectum mucosa (rectal membrane) at such a time to assist dilation of the rectum in being ready to perform this action.

  Typical dis-ease Piles or mucus in the stools.

> *Based on the perceived stressor, the body will process a metaphorical interpretation by way of response and will adapt on a cellular level to compensate and to assist in resolving the issue."*

The purpose of the biological adaptation in each case is to facilitate resolution of the problem: I cannot digest this situation so I will increase my digestive ability; I cannot face other people so I need to be thicker-skinned; I am not strong enough to confront authority so I must be stronger; I cannot define my position so I need to make my position clear.

Based on the perceived stressor, the body will process a metaphorical interpretation by way of response and will adapt on a cellular level to compensate and to assist in resolving the issue. These short bio-logical programmes are happening all the time without our awareness. However, if these programmes are over-stimulated, problems can occur in our biological responses. The body makes a slight adaptation to deal with the instant event, but if you get stuck in a thought, the body may be stimulated to do so again and again. This can be the beginning of dis-ease, commonly known as illness.

E - Emotional

To understand why we get stuck in a bio-logical programme, it would help to understand what part our emotions play in the process.

There are many philosophies and studies of emotions but, put simply, some of our emotions have a positive influence on the body - like joy, happiness, love and appreciation - while other emotions have a negative impact on the body - such as anger, sadness, fear, worry, disgust, guilt and jealously. None of these emotions is detrimental to our health in themselves. It is when we cannot process an emotion that we trigger an adaptation in the body that may give rise to a symptom of dis-ease.

What are emotions? Emotions are literally energy-in-motion. They are energetic messages sent around the body - we might even call them 'e-motions'. They relay information faster than chemical messages and can be identified as sensations in the energetic system. For example, if I were to ask you to imagine standing on a stage in front of three thousand people to recite Shakespeare's *Hamlet*, where would you feel that in your body? It doesn't matter whether you might be excited, nervous or petrified, the emotion you would have is an energetic response. If you imagine answering the door to a stranger to have him barge into your house uninvited, where do you feel that in your body? It could be fear, anger, confusion - that emotion expresses itself as a certain kind of sensation. Emotion is the connection between your thoughts and how they are felt in your body.

Event/perception > e-motion > bodily response.

Perceiving danger

Our perceptions of what may be dangerous or a threat to us are linked to our deepest, fundamental need for survival. This need extends to being accepted (for if I am alone, I might die) and to be loved (if I am unloved, I am alone and cast out and I might die). If we explore any emotion, however negative it may appear, we will find beneath the desire to be loved, accepted and appreciated, or perhaps more explicitly, the fear of being unloved, unaccepted and unappreciated. So why do some people have more negative emotions than others?

We all may experience trauma in our life at some time - the loss of a loved one, divorce, an accident, an attack, loss of a job. However, our beliefs and perceptions, and therefore our ability to handle these life traumas, are formed when we are much younger - by the time we are six years' old in fact. This is because during this period of our life we are in a highly receptive brain state. Our adult brains are usually in one of four brainwave states.

Brainwave states

- **Beta** Normal, adult active-thinking (13-30 Hz)
- **Alpha** Meditation, praying, light hypnotic trance, waking or falling asleep (8-12 Hz)
- **Theta** Deep hypnotic trance, dreaming (4-8 Hz)
- **Delta** Deep sleep, normal infant state (less than 4 Hz)

Babies spend the first two years of life in a constant *delta* brainwave state – a kind of sleep state.

Between the ages of two- and approximately six years' old, children are in the *theta* state – as in a waking dream. Therefore, young children are in a deep hypnagogic trance and absorb everything around them like a sponge. Nature does this so that we can download at a rapid rate all the survival information we need for life. So, we learn everything by seeing and copying until the age of six years' old. It is during this time also that we form our view of ourselves and the world around us. This view is largely inherited from our parents and our primary careers, but also from other family members, authority figures and the media. We begin this learning process when we are still in the womb and continue to download information as survival guidelines throughout those first six years. To a child, everything it learns is a truth by which it will make sense of the world later, even if this apparent 'truth' is in fact a misinterpretation.

This means that the child who has lived with more danger will adapt to be prepared for danger. The child who was taught that they were always wrong will believe that they cannot get anything right and the child that watched his parents being violent when they were upset will grow up with violence issues, either acting violently or expecting to be treated in such a way. This gives rise to very individual perceptions of the same event by different people.

Did the thought of someone barging into your house make you feel afraid or angry? Where did you learn to feel that? We model what we learned as a child and do not usually question how we react or how we feel. This is even the case when we are unhappy with our feelings and our emotional, psychological or physical health. We still don't question where our unhappiness came from, because it's real to us.

As an energy therapist, I work with people to change their responses by evolving and releasing their emotions. Emotional energy gets stuck in your energetic system and, unless it is released, you can become trapped in a loop of thoughts and limiting beliefs. This in turn sends messages to your body to continue responding, preventing a return to health. There is a direct relationship between the thought, the feeling and the physical symptom. Working with this connection allows you to evolve the energy and change the thought processes, thus allowing the body to return to health.

T – Tissue

Every tissue in the body has a unique job to perform. Every cell is formed of proteins assembled in such a way as to carry out a specific function. These cells work together to form tissues, organs and systems. All these systems, and the human body as a whole, work to a perfect, original blueprint. This exquisite design, the template by which the body is organised and structured, may be seen in the detail of the tissue, where each cell performs its unique function.

We can examine the function of the tissue and relate it to its corresponding brain layer. This gives us some insight into the perception and emotional response that might trigger an adaptation in the working of a particular tissue cell.

The kidney is a good example of how different tissues within one organ have different jobs. The kidney is formed from tissues that originate from three different germ layers, which means that they are associated with three different brain layers with different themes. This also means that each of these tissues reacts in a unique way in an attempt to resolve a specific issue. Each tissue is triggered into a specific response by a different trauma or trigger.

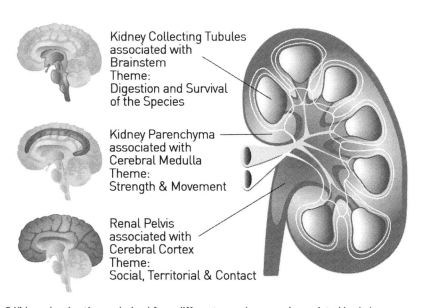

Kidney Collecting Tubules associated with Brainstem
Theme:
Digestion and Survival of the Species

Kidney Parenchyma associated with Cerebral Medulla
Theme:
Strength & Movement

Renal Pelvis associated with Cerebral Cortex
Theme:
Social, Territorial & Contact

Fig.5 Kidney showing tissues derived from different germ layers and associated brain layers

The kidney's main function is to filter and clean the blood and to remove and pass waste water to the bladder. The different parts of the kidney support that process with separate functions. The following triggers in our daily perception of events may set off corresponding bio-logical responses in different parts of the kidney.

Kidney collecting tubules

- Function: to regulate water retention
- Tissue: endoderm
- Brain layer: brainstem
- Theme: digestion and survival of species
- Trigger: feelings of isolation, abandonment, or being deserted.

Kidney parenchyma

- Function: to filter and remove waste water
- Tissue: mesoderm
- Brain layer: cerebral medulla
- Theme: movement and strength
- Trigger: fear of drowning or fearful experience around water or liquid.

Renal pelvis

- Function: to collect waste water to pass to the bladder
- Tissue: ectoderm
- Brain layer: cerebral cortex
- Theme: social, territorial, contact
- Trigger: unable to define or mark territory or not knowing what position to take.

A – Adaptation

Every tissue in the body has the capacity to adapt to compensate and regulate the bodily processes to aid in its defence. The body is designed to be adaptive and to cope with day-to-day shifts and changes. However, these changes are not meant to be long term - they are brief programmes to adjust to short-term stressors. Once triggered, the tissue is supposed only to adapt, with an increase or decrease of cells, for a short time, until the stress has passed and equilibrium is restored. The aim of the body is always to return to health and balance, to normal function.

> ❝ *The aim of the body is always to return to health and balance, to normal function.*❞

The original bio-logical purpose of the organ tissue adaptation is fundamentally animalistic, but it can also be stimulated by a misperception or a belief. The body will still respond to the signal and adapt accordingly. This means that an unresolved issue or a deep belief can re-trigger a programme so that the tissue continues to respond.

If continually stimulated in this way, the tissue will continue to adapt to the problem, in an attempt to meet the strain on the system imposed by the stressor, even if the stressor is not an actual one, but the memory or fear of one. This constant re-triggering can result in dis-ease.

Now let us look again at our examples to see the bio-logical purpose of these adaptations:

Kidney collecting tubules

- Function: to regulate water retention
- Tissue: endoderm
- Brain layer: brainstem
- Theme: digestion and survival
- Trigger: feelings of isolation and abandonment
- Purpose of the bio-logical tissue adaptation: apart from oxygen, water is the most important thing for survival. When one is separated from the flock and in danger of being left alone and unable to find food and water, the body adjusts by retaining more water and storing it in the body. This is a fundamental survival technique triggered in animals when separated. In modern society, we may not be far from water, but the body responds to a metaphoric

58

threat to survival if the person feels isolated, abandoned, alone or disconnected from others. Someone experiencing emotions on this theme would trigger this programme and retain water.

Kidney parenchyma

- Function: to filter and remove waste-water
- Tissue: mesoderm
- Brain layer: cerebral medulla
- Theme: movement and strength
- Trigger: fear of drowning or fearful experience around water or liquid
- Purpose of the bio-logical tissue adaptation: the kidney cleans the blood and removes water and waste from the system. When triggered by a fear around water, the body will begin a programme aimed at being stronger and better at processing water from the body.

Renal pelvis

- Function: to collect waste-water to pass to bladder
- Tissue: ectoderm
- Brain layer: cerebral cortex
- Theme: social, territorial, contact
- Trigger: unable to define or mark territory or not knowing what position to take
- Purpose of the bio-logical tissue adaptation: there is an ulcerative dilation of the renal pelvis in order to pass urine more quickly to the urethra and down towards the bladder for territory marking.

In each of these examples, we can see that a real event, a memory or fear of a future event can trigger the tissue to respond. If this were a fleeting adaptation, we would not necessarily notice the change, or perhaps only have passing symptoms as the body adjusts to continue its function under a changing load. When the message is sent repeatedly or inappropriately to the organ, however, the tissue will continue to respond and, in time, can cause disease. Unless we understand this connection, the reason for the change, it is difficult to get to the root cause of the disease and we are left to manage symptoms.

When we know what the symptoms represent and can understand the activity as a particular bio-logical function, we can identify the traumatic event or trigger that instigates the adaptation.

The tissue function and order

Each of the tissues in the body responds in a different way according to the germ layer from which it derived and the brain layer to which it corresponds. We know that tissue derived from ectoderm, which is associated with the brainstem, and tissues derived from old mesoderm, associated with the cerebellum, both increase their cell numbers when triggered by a stressful event or thought. Tissues that derive from the new mesoderm, associated with the cerebral medulla, and tissue derived from ectoderm, associated with the cerebral cortex, on the other hand show a decrease in cell numbers when triggered by a stressful event or thought.

Depending on the function of the organ tissue, an increase or decrease of cells is necessary to improve function during a time of stress.

Brainstem - increase of cells

For tissues associated with the brainstem (theme: digestion and survival of the species), we see an increase in cells when triggered by a stressor to help the tissue in the organ to perform its task better.

For example, in the liver an increase in cells would improve the uptake of nutrients from food. It would be triggered by a fear of starving or 'not knowing where the next meal is coming from'. This could even extend to a more metaphoric starvation, such as 'not enough love for me', as in the case of one client.

Cerebellum - increase of cells

For tissues associated with the cerebellum (theme: protection and integrity), we see an increase in cells, when triggered by a stressor, in order to form thicker barriers or buffers, to protect against an impending attack. For example, a thickening of the peritoneum, the protective lining in the abdominal cavity, would support and protect the abdominal organs. It would be triggered by a direct attack to the abdomen, but could also be triggered by a traumatic event received like 'a kick in the guts'.

Cerebral medulla - decrease of cells

For tissue associated with the cerebral medulla (theme: movement and strength), such as bones, muscles, tendons, ligaments and the lymph system, we see a decrease in cells when triggered by a stressor and therefore a reduction of tissue. The cerebral medulla is unique in that it must complete two parts of a programme to fulfil its biological purpose: there is a weakening, followed by a strengthening of the tissue, resulting in a stronger tissue than before.

Cerebral cortex - decrease of cells

For tissues associated with the cerebral cortex (theme: social, territorial and personal contact), we see a decrease in cells when triggered by a stressor to create an ulcerative effect, which is a thinning of the lining of part of the organ. This thinning of the tissue allows for a dilation of the passageways to create space for a fuller or easier flow of substances such as blood, water and food. It could also be the thinning of the epidermis of the skin, which causes a desensitisation to touch.

Perception and response to threat

When we perceive a threat, a mechanism called the 'fight or flight response' is alerted to focus our energies into the parts of the body that are required for flight or, if we can't flee, to fight. When we sense an imminent threat to our survival, which could be through hearing, seeing, smelling, tasting or feeling something, a response is triggered in the body. We experience it as a spontaneous reaction to the perception, but in fact a very complex process has been activated.

6 6 *When we sense an imminent threat to our survival, which could be through hearing, seeing, smelling, tasting or feeling something, a response is triggered in the body. We experience it as a spontaneous reaction to the perception, but in fact a very complex process has been activated.* "

The day-to-day function of your body goes on without your conscious knowledge. Your circulation, heart rate, digestion, breathing, perspiration - indeed, all your organs - are controlled by the autonomic nervous system, the control system run by the subconscious. The 'fight or flight' mechanism effectively hijacks the autonomic nervous system, flooding it with hormones that prime the body for reaction. Hormones from the pituitary and adrenal glands trigger the release of cortisol (often called the stress hormone), which in turn increases blood pressure, blood sugar and suppresses the immune system. Blood is diverted from the digestive system and the extremities to the major muscles, in order to prioritise action or escape - this is no time to be digesting! When faced with an uncomfortable situation that makes you nervous - such as a confrontation - the funny 'butterflies' feeling you get in your tummy is the blood moving from the intestines to the main muscles so that you can respond. When we go into the 'stress' response, we also often experience cold hands and feet and go pale, because there is no need for blood in the extremities and it is prioritised for the muscles.

The 'freeze' response is the third way we cope when faced with helplessness and a threat to survival. Our response is initially to flee; if we cannot flee, we are primed to fight, but if this is not an option we will freeze.

Most specialists who deal with trauma and stress still work within the paradigm of the current medical model that sees illnesses as a mistake or malfunction of the body. As a result, there has been much research into the effects of stress on the HPA axis[23], which constitutes a major part of the neuroendocrine system controlling and regulating many body processes, including digestion, the immune system, mood and emotions, sexuality and energy storage and expenditure. At the same time, there has been little connection between this research and the META-Health understanding of individual organ responses that occur at the same time as the HPA-axis response. As well as the response of the limbic system, there is a separate and dedicated organ response that helps to process the threat and makes an adjustment in that organ to compensate for it.

For example, the fear that someone will enter or leave your territory beyond your control will trigger the panic of a fight or flight response, but, if you are unable to respond, you will also create a response in the bronchial mucous membranes. The membranes will immediately thin to widen the bronchial tubes and allow the passage of more air so that you can face up to the situation. With this trigger, you do not feel a physical symptom because your airflow is easier, in order to cope with the situation. Once the danger has passed, however, the bronchial membranes must rest, repair and replenish and this results in a restriction in the bronchial tubes (causing shortness of breath, chesty cough or asthma).

This example demonstrates the need to understand the next important META principle of the two phases of dis-ease.

When you have symptoms, you may be in stress, but as with the example of the bronchial mucous membranes, you may have entered into a state of rest and repair, during which your symptoms are present while repair of the tissue takes place. Knowing at what stage you are during a process of stress and repair is important in being able to identify what to do to resolve the issue and to be able to support the body back to health.

---

23 'The **hypothalamic-pituitary-adrenal axis (HPA or HTPA axis)**, also known as the **limbic-hypothalamic-pituitary-adrenal axis** (LHPA axis)'. (Wikipedia)

4. Your disease is not a life sentence

"Cells respond to a massive variety of signals using protein switches: over 100,000 switches per cell built into its membrane. These protein switches are fundamental units of perception. They read environmental conditions and adjust the biology to meet the need required. This becomes very profound when we own that perception controls behavior, for it is how we perceive the world that controls our lives.'

Dr Bruce Lipton[24]

When faced with a threat, you are able immediately to prioritise the most effective method for your survival. Your first choice is to run away or for flight, so you instinctively assess the escape options. If no escape is possible, or when you are in a social situation where running away is not an option, your second priority is to fight. If this too is not an option - for example a gazelle cannot fight a lion and, at work, you do not normally fight your boss - the third option is to freeze. If you adopt the 'freeze' response, this will require a different reaction within the nervous system: instead of gearing up for action, the heart rate and responses slow.

Your body is always seeking harmony and balance. Health is a state of balance and flow. When triggered by a stressor, your body receives a message and is stimulated to compensate for the stressful event or situation. This involves a specific organ response that happens in synchronicity with the fight/flight/ freeze mechanism. As soon as the threat has passed, the body will complete the process and go into a state of repair before it returns to equilibrium.

---

24 *The Biology of Belief - Unleashing the Power of Consciousness, Matter & Miracles*, Bruce H. Lipton PhD, op. cit.

It is always the case that there are two phases to every illness or dis-ease in the body. There is a stress phase, which begins immediately the threat occurs, and a regeneration phase, when repair takes place and balance is restored once the threat has passed. All diseases go through these two phases and every tissue responds in a specific way during the stress phase and subsequently in the regeneration phase.

The natural laws of balance

Balance is not stagnant. By its nature, energy must flow and balance is ever-changing and forever re-establishing itself. Our ability to maintain a healthy balance lies in our ability to recover and to allow energy to flow again. A balanced energy system is able to maintain a state of flow, processing energy received in such a way as to manage its flow through and from the system. The Chinese Yin/Yang symbol describes how apparently opposite dualities – light/dark, water/fire, life/death – interact with one another to create a greater, indivisible harmony. So too in our energy flow there is no good or bad energy: there is just the need for balance.

In the stress phase, we usually have obsessive thoughts about how to solve the problem that is stressing us. We run scenarios in our head and, if we have a number of issues that are active at the same time, we can become very distracted. We are more hyperactive and often have less appetite and may lose weight. We do not sleep well when we go to bed and can wake at odd hours. This stress phase is often called the 'cold phase', because blood is diverted to the muscles to prepare us for 'fight or flight' action, thus de-prioritising supply to the digestive system and the extremities, which become cold.

Authorities such as Dr Bruce Lipton[25] and Dr Robert Scaer[26] remind us that the body cannot be both in a state of 'fight or flight' and in a state of 'rest and repair' at the same time. This makes bio-logical sense, because it is clearly no good to be calmly licking your wounds or digesting your dinner

---

25 The Biology of Belief – Unleashing the Power of Consciousness, Matter & Miracles, Bruce H. Lipton PhD, op. cit.
26 The Body Bears the Burden – Trauma, Dissociation and Disease (2nd ed.), Robert C. Scaer MD, op. cit.

if a big tiger is about to devour you! You must first escape the tiger. Only then does it make sense to rest, nurse your wounds, repair damage done - and digest your dinner!

The amount of stress put on a system in the first (stress) phase must be compensated for in the second (rest and repair) phase. If the stress has been particularly severe or prolonged, it is possible to experience strong reactions during the repair phase in the attempt to restore balance. Imagine a pendulum that has been forced to swing very high in one direction; it must first swing back the other way almost as high before it can settle back to the centre. By the same token, the intensity of the trauma while the tiger chased you must be released, after the danger has passed, by an equally intense process of repair.

If a traumatic event is so great that we put massive stress into the system, it will certainly create a great impact. Equally, however, if we continually re-trigger a series of smaller traumatic events on a regular basis, we can similarly increase the stress load on the brain and the associated organs. If stress is not processed as it arises, we store it in our memories and thoughts and replay them in our heads in search of resolution. We also maintain a sensory awareness so that we can scan for possible future traumas and we live with the process still active in our systems. All these processes of unresolved stress and trauma remain active, but largely unconscious to us.

If you are unhappy with a situation or limitation in your life, habits or patterns that hold you back from doing what you want to do, or if you have psychological or physical issues that you don't seem able to resolve, you are probably stuck in past thoughts and beliefs, based on what you learned from your past traumas. These could be big traumas or the small traumas and events you experience before the age of six, when you were making sense of the world. In this way, it is possible to decode the symptoms of disease to build a picture of what you are experiencing or have experienced in your life that has led to becoming unwell. Information from the symptoms takes you back to the root cause of the problem - the pattern of triggers and the original trauma. It is of course possible to have a traumatic experience at any time in life, but your pattern for handling trauma and stressful events is already in place as a result of your early experiences and understanding of yourself and the world. This is why I refer to pre-six years' old as being a significant period to investigate.

A healthy response

It is important to remember that the response that the body has to a threat is initially a healthy one. It is specifically designed to cope with emergencies - as in the case of a tiger. If the threat is real and transitory, the body is able to compensate for a short period before entering the repair phase where balance is restored.

> *The amount of stress put on a system in the first (stress) phase must be compensated for in the second (rest and repair) phase. If the stress has been particularly severe or prolonged, it is possible to experience strong reactions during the repair phase in the attempt to restore balance.*

Imagine a rabbit chased by a fox. A number of physiological adaptations need to occur very quickly for the rabbit to escape. His heart needs to pump faster; his muscles need to work more quickly for him to flee; he needs to get more oxygen into his system to help him escape. Once the rabbit has escaped and is safe, he can rest. His heart rate and breathing will normalise; his muscles and nerves will repair. In fact, most of his system will repair stronger than before so that he can be even faster next time to avoid capture.

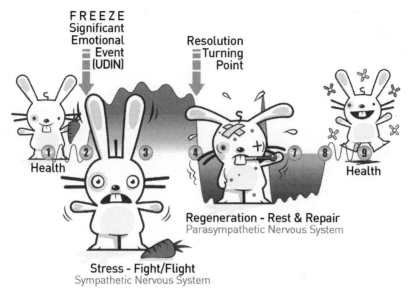

FREEZE
Significant
Emotional
Event
(UDIN)

Resolution
Turning
Point

Health

Health

Regeneration - Rest & Repair
Parasympathetic Nervous System

Stress - Fight/Flight
Sympathetic Nervous System

Fig.6 The rabbits fight / flight / freeze response to danger, followed by regeneration, rest and repair

Releasing the freeze

An important aspect of the rabbit's experience is that he will release the trauma from his system and enter quickly into repairing the changes in his body. After his repair, however, he will return to his daily habits again. He has a natural instinct to be aware of danger, but, once he has released the trauma, he does not keep re-living it, neither does he 'plan' for the next incident.

All animals in the wild process their life-threatening events. If an animal in the wild cannot flee or fight and enters into a freeze response, its natural instinct is to shake as soon as the danger passes, in order to release the build-up of energy in the system and return to equilibrium. Unfortunately, because of social constraints, we humans do not release our freeze responses, but hold onto the trauma within our systems. This is also true of domestic and caged animals.

The wild rabbit processed the trauma in what is called 'procedural memory', which subconsciously acts out the event being resolved. If we were to observe the rabbit at this point, we would see it acting out the running away from

69

danger that it was unable to do before the freeze response kicked in. The release of this trauma usually involves a shaking or trembling and a running motion, while the energy of the trauma is released from the rabbit's system. The energy of the event is released along with all the build-up of chemicals and tension. Although it is capable of responding should the same event happen again, the rabbit is not constantly living in fear that the fox is going to enter its territory and eat it. People who don't let go of their trauma, on the other hand, may exhibit a whole range of resulting dis-eases. A fear of someone entering your territory, for example, would trigger the bronchial mucous membranes to respond and make the bronchial airways temporarily wider to allow in more oxygen. If that freeze is not released, the circumstances of the event are likely to be re-triggered because the response process has not been completed. This leads the body to continue to respond, creating ongoing dis-eases such as bronchitis or asthma.

Wild bunnies don't get asthma!

Coping with challenge or change

It is natural to face challenges or changes and we must have some mechanism to manage the fluctuation of demands on our mental, physical and emotional resources. Ensuring that we have enough rest is certainly important; a healthy diet and exercise maintain our systems; so too do healthy emotional outlooks. If we are easily triggered into stress, we run the risk of depleting our resources and of remaining stuck in incomplete programmes that become detrimental to our health. If the rabbit had escaped, but did not release his freeze and instead formed a belief that he was not quick enough to escape in future, or that the fox was always waiting round the corner to pounce on him, he would become stuck in a programme and would begin to show signs of stress dis-ease:

- **Bunny belief** - *I will be attacked from behind.*

  Programme - I need to not look behind, but to focus on my escape route.

Bio-logical purpose - There is a reduction in the retinal and peripheral vision.

Resulting dis-ease - If repeatedly re-triggered, it will result in myopia, tunnel vision or loss of sight.

- **Bunny belief** - *The fox is going to come back and get me.*

  Programme - I need to take in more oxygen quickly to face up to the attack, resulting in a thinning of the mucous membranes.

  Biological purpose - The thinning of the membranes widens the bronchial tubes to allow more air in.

  Resulting dis-ease - Bronchitis or asthma (stuck in second phase, constantly repairing the tissue so the airways are clogged up).

Wild animals that release the freeze can quickly go about their business and return to normal psychological and physiological function. It is the inability to flee, fight or release the freeze response, that is, to have any form of resolution and processing of the event that results in an ongoing, inappropriate response to the situation.

Nature's two phases of disease

It is important to know what happens to individual tissues in the first and second stress phases. It is also important to know what keeps a person stuck in one or the other phase, so that we can understand what symptoms may occur as a result.

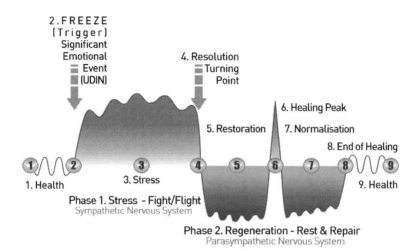

Fig.7 The 9 points and two phases of dis-ease used in META-Health analysis

In the diagram above, we can see nine points in the dis-ease process.

1. Normal health - no trauma or stress.
2. The traumatic event (or the re-triggering thought or stimulus) that we refer to as the UDIN (Unexpected, Dramatic, Isolating and No strategy to cope) or SEE (Significant Emotional Event).
3. The first (stress) phase – where there is a change in the tissue(s) of the relevant organ(s), together with obsessive thinking and an agitated response because of the fight or flight mechanism. This is known as the 'cold phase', because the extremities become cold when the blood flow is prioritised for the muscles. The blood also moves from the digestive system, so during this phase there is usually no appetite and digestion is not active.
4. The resolution – the turning point at which the threatening situation is resolved, either by the danger being evaded or through a change in perception of the danger, for example realising that the situation is not life-threatening after all.

5. The first part of the regeneration phase –this is when repair to the organ tissue takes place. There is usually oedema[27] (water-retention) and swelling; this is the stage at which fungi, mycobacteria, bacteria or viruses may become engaged.

6. The 'healing peak', when the organ no longer needs the extra water and can push this out of the organ and the system. At this point, there is also a dip back into the stress phase, including a psychological revisit of the traumatic situation.

7. The second part of the regeneration phase – this stage involves normalising the usual function of the organ and a return to health.

8. Completion of the full programme.

9. Return to health.

The two phases of dis-ease

Here we can see how the two phases of dis-ease balance out. From the first point of the trauma or trigger, we enter into the stress phase and the tissue makes an adaptation. Depending on the tissue and its function, it will react in one of two ways: either with an increase or decrease of cells, whichever will increase organ function during stress.

Let us look at an example of what happens in the first and second phase for each of the brain layers:

*   **Tissue associated with the brainstem**

    Increase of cells in the tonsils

    Stress trigger, first phase - Inability to swallow or let go of something, like having the taste of something then having it snatched away or having something that you need to get out but can't.

---

27 **Oedema** 'is an abnormal accumulation of fluid in the interstitium, which are locations beneath the skin or in one or more cavities of the body. It is clinically shown as swelling.' (Wikipedia)

Tissue reaction - Enlargement of the pharyngeal tonsil (adenoid) as more cells are made to assist with grasping or holding onto the 'chunk'.

This 'chunk' does not have to be food, but can be information, such as being promised something - to have a taste for it, but then have it taken away.

Example - *A nine-year-old girl, Chloe, was on a strict diet of health food and was not allowed things such as chocolate and ice cream. Chloe was sure she would be allowed an ice cream with her friends, but was not and had to watch her friends eat ice cream and could imagine what it would taste like to eat. She was very upset at not being able to enjoy the same foods as her friends and developed swollen tonsils.*

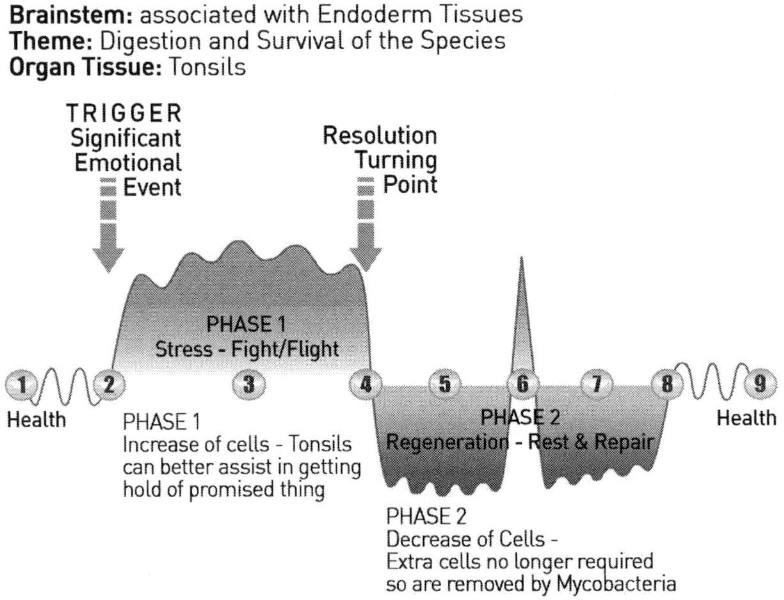

Brainstem: associated with Endoderm Tissues
Theme: Digestion and Survival of the Species
Organ Tissue: Tonsils

Fig.8 The response of the tissue of the tonsils throughout the two phases of dis-ease

Regeneration trigger, turning point into second phase - Chloe was able to negotiate with her mother to have a different, more appropriate treat. She resolved the emotional issue and was no longer upset about the ice cream. In the second phase, Chloe's tonsils, which had swollen, began to eliminate the extra cells with the help of *Mycobacterium tuberculosis*. This appears as an infection and is commonly known as tonsillitis.

- **Tissue associated with the cerebellum**

Increase of cells in mammary (breast) tissue

Stress trigger, first phase - Fear and worry with regard to an argument or conflict in the 'nest'. This can be with one's mate, father, mother, child or about the home itself - the nest.

Tissue reaction - An increase in mammary-gland cells, based on the perception that it is the woman's biological job to tend the nest, provide milk and to nurture and take care of the family and children. The cell increase in the breast tissue (the lobules) increases the woman's ability to make milk, thus increasing her capacity for nurturing and providing sustenance.

Example - *A lady in her thirties, Emma, was unhappy at home and considering leaving, but her friend talked her into staying, by explaining that marriage was hard work and you had to stick at it. Emma stayed, despite all the arguing and unhappiness, and developed a tumour in her right breast.*

Regeneration trigger, turning point into second phase - For Emma, there was no emotional resolution and so no turning point in the two phases, which meant that she stayed fixed in the first (stress) phase. She chose to go for surgery to have the tumour removed. However, the illness did change the relationship between her and her husband, who became more supportive of her because of her illness.

If Emma had resolved her issue by changing her situation or changing how she felt about the situation, she would have seen a decrease in her mammary tissue with *Mycobacterium tuberculosis* helping to degrade the tissue.

This engagement of fungi, bacteria and viruses is a very different concept of healing to the current medical model. I encourage you to weigh up the notion that nasty bugs are attacking us against the idea that those microbes are symbiotically co-operating within a balanced ecosystem. Where there are severe symptoms of microbe activity, it is true it can be a difficult, uncomfortable and unpleasant experience. However, the amount of activity will be in direct proportion to the amount of stress and therefore the amount of repair required - this counterbalancing effect is the key determining factor.

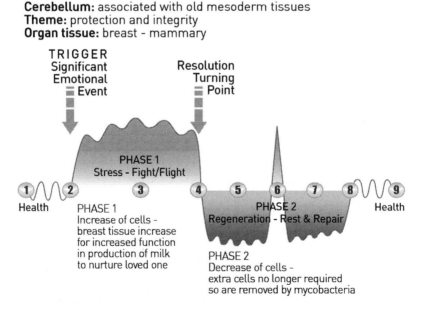

Cerebellum: associated with old mesoderm tissues
Theme: protection and integrity
Organ tissue: breast - mammary

TRIGGER
Significant
Emotional
Event

Resolution
Turning
Point

PHASE 1
Stress - Fight/Flight

Health

PHASE 1
Increase of cells -
breast tissue increase
for increased function
in production of milk
to nurture loved one

PHASE 2
Regeneration - Rest & Repair

Health

PHASE 2
Decrease of cells -
extra cells no longer required
so are removed by mycobacteria

Fig.9 The response of the tissues of the breast (mammary) gland throughout the two phases of dis-ease

Cerebral Medulla: associated with New Mesoderm Tissues
Theme: Movement and Strength
Organ Tissue: Knee - Bone, Cartilage, Muscle

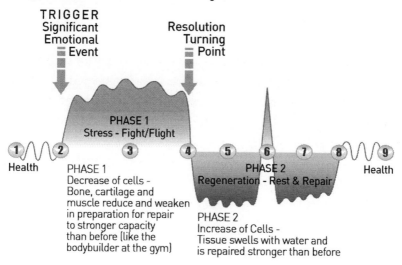

Fig. 10 The response of the tissue of the knee bone, cartilage and muscle throughout the two phases of dis-ease

- **Tissue associated with the cerebral medulla**

Decrease of cells in the knee-joint tissue

Stress trigger, first phase - Not being strong enough to compete or move forwards in a situation or relationship.

Tissue reaction - Tissues associated with the cerebral medulla are unique in that they need to go through both the stress phase (in which there is a decrease in cells and therefore a weakening of muscles, bones and joints) *and* through the regeneration phase (during which the cells are replenished and tissue repaired, so that the organ can be stronger for next time).

Example - *Eric felt that he could not compete with other, younger men who did the same job as him. He was worried that they were better than him and that he would not be able to keep up with them*

77

and attract clients. This affected his self-esteem and he took up sport to 'get fit' and to feel better about himself.

Regeneration trigger, turning point into second phase - Because Eric had felt 'not strong enough to compete', doing something that made him feel fitter and stronger made him feel better about himself. This resolved his emotional issue and took him into the second phase, where his tissue could regenerate and become stronger.

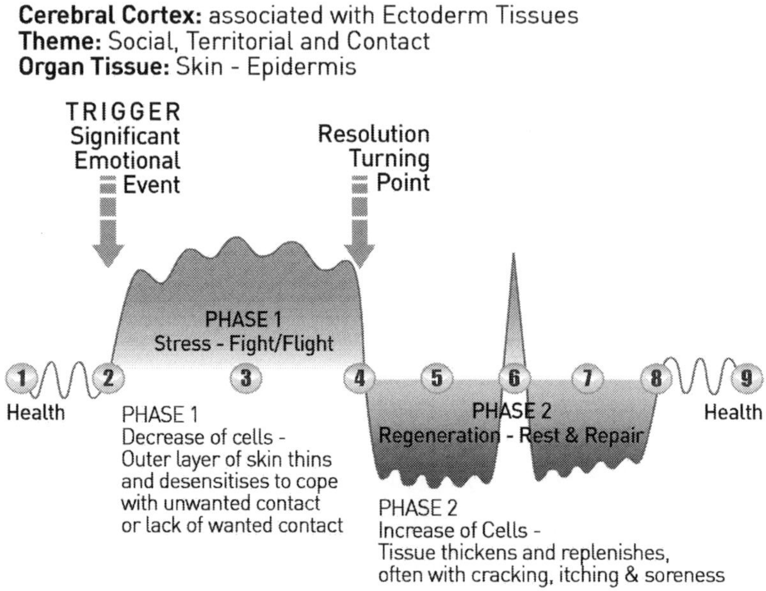

Cerebral Cortex: associated with Ectoderm Tissues
Theme: Social, Territorial and Contact
Organ Tissue: Skin - Epidermis

Fig.11 The response of the outer layer of the skin (epidermis) throughout the two phases of dis-ease

- **Tissue associated with the cerebral cortex**

Decrease of cells in the epidermis of the skin

Stress trigger, first phase - Either unwanted contact that you don't want to feel (such as from a person who repels you for some reason)

78

or contact that you do want to feel, but can't have (such as someone whose touch you long for, but can't have because they are not willing to touch you or because there has been a separation of some kind).

Tissue reaction - In both cases, the epidermis of the skin thins and desensitises in order to reduce the need to feel contact. In the case of unwanted contact, it occurs to avoid being reminded of the touch. In the case of a lack of wanted contact, it allows us to cope better with missing or needing the touch, for example 'if I can't feel, I will not miss the contact.'

Example - *Alice, a lady in her mid-fifties, experienced a thinning of the skin on the palms of her hands. She had wanted to hold onto her estranged brother and missed being able to touch and hold him. He also represented contact with the rest of her family.*

Regeneration trigger, turning point into second phase - Alice did some work on her emotions about missing her family and not having contact with her brother. She released some of the trauma of feeling separated and was able to progress into the regeneration phase. In the second phase, the symptoms of eczema occur as the skin replenishes cells and sensitivity returns.

The important aspect here is that there is a process. Once the healing has occurred, the body will return to a balanced state of health. Although resolving the issue will initially bring symptoms of eczema, this phase need last only as long as the body needs to heal the tissue. Ongoing health problems are caused by a re-triggering of the original trauma response. This is why it is important to release the trauma.

A balanced ecosystem

By examining what happens in both phases, we are forced to examine a concept in META-Health that is very different to the standard medical interpretation and can be somewhat controversial – the body's relationship with fungi, mycobacteria, bacteria and viruses.

For me this has been one of the biggest breakthroughs in changing my perspective when I have an illness. I nurture my body through the incubation period, allowing the bacteria or virus to do its work during rest and repair so that my body can heal and replenish. The engaged microbes are either assisting in repairing the tissue, or are breaking down tissue that is no longer required. This is a process that must be fully traversed in order to return to health and balance.

Because our experiences with fungi, bacteria, mycobacteria and viruses are seldom pleasant, it is a challenging step to consider that the things we have always believed to be attacking us could possibly be working with our bodies to do a specific job. Let us not forget that the largest part of pharmaceutical companies' income is made by selling drugs that eradicate 'pathogens' that attack us and are seen as the causes of disease. In META-Health we do not differentiate between good and bad bacteria - there are just bacteria that may or may not be engaged by your body in a dis-ease process.

When bacteria are active, we can have symptoms that are very unpleasant and we feel unwell, often with fever. So how can we consider this to be part of a helpful process?

Let's first be clear that we are not denying that fungi, mycobacteria, bacteria and viruses are present and active during the symptoms of dis-ease. The different perspective I am offering is that, even if their activity is the cause of the symptoms, they are *not the original cause of the problem*. They are bio-logical helpers and perform a vital function. They are required to bring the body back into balance.

The little boy and the fire

A little boy was out with his father one morning and they passed a house on fire. There was much activity as the firemen battled with the blaze to extinguish it. 'Daddy, how are fires caused?' asked the little boy, curious about all the commotion. 'I don't know, son', replied the father.

Some time later, the little boy was out with his father again and they passed a shop that was on fire, again with fireman bravely rushing around with hoses and ladders extinguishing the fire. 'Daddy, how are fires caused?' asked the boy again. Again the father replied, 'I don't know, son.'

> *Is it at all possible that we have been misinterpreting the role of fungi, mycobacteria, bacteria and viruses in their presence and function – simply because they are 'always there' when illness is present?"*

On yet a third occasion, the boy and his father saw another building blazing fiercely, with fire engines, firemen on ladders and with hoses, water and foam everywhere. Before the boy could ask again, the father said, 'I am sorry, son, I don't know how fires are caused.' This time the boy smiled and said, 'Oh, it's OK, Daddy, I know how fires are caused. It must be those big red engines and those firemen, because every time there is a fire, they are always there!'

Is it at all possible that we have been misinterpreting the role of fungi, mycobacteria, bacteria and viruses in their presence and function – simply because they are 'always there' when illness is present?

Let us come back to our example of tonsillitis.

In her stress phase, Chloe had swollen tonsils while there was an increase of cells to better hold onto the desired morsel.

In this case, the mycobacteria were not active during the first (stress) phase. There would be mycobacteria in Chloe's system awaiting a trigger to become active and to take away the extra tonsil tissue - unless of course Chloe had taken antibiotics to kill them and clear them from her system. If left to perform their natural process, each cell will be ready and waiting to perform its function as soon as the second phase is entered into and the extra cells can be removed. This is an incredibly intelligent process!

When the issue is resolved, the mycobacteria would be engaged and the extra tonsil tissue broken down and digested by them. In this phase, we see the full symptoms of tonsillitis. The seriousness of the symptoms in the second phase will be proportionate to the amount of stress in the first (stress) phase. The greater the emotional stress about the initial issue, the more serious will be the bout of tonsillitis. This would also be the case if there were an ongoing trigger, in which the issue kept repeating and building up unresolved stress.

If Chloe did not have the mycobacteria to degrade her tonsil tissue, she would be left with enlarged tonsils and, if the issue were to repeat, her symptoms would be more pronounced in the stress phase. On the other hand, if Chloe had resolved her issue but didn't have the right bacteria in her body to complete the repair process, she might be lucky enough to catch the mycobacterium from a child at school and then be able to enter into the second phase in which the bacteria would help with tissue breakdown and repair. This goes some way to explain how we 'catch colds'.

I appreciate that this opens up a whole can of worms regarding our existing belief systems and challenges a globally adopted concept that creates very good business! It also takes us into discussions about epidemics and immunisation that are all exciting food for thought – if you want to break out of the existing paradigm of being a victim to things that 'happen to you' beyond your control, rather than being part of a balanced ecosystem.

When we look at returning to health, we should also take into account the threshold of health that each individual possesses. We also need to bear in mind that the amount of stress that is put into the system has to be handled by the system, processed and released, before the person can begin to feel better. This can lead to great imbalances and severe symptoms in one of the, or sometimes in both, phases of dis-ease. Some fungal, bacterial and viral activity can cause fatality and disease certainly needs to be managed very carefully, with the help of doctors and sometimes appropriate medications and interventions.

It is also helpful to both doctor and patient to understand what process is at work and to remember that any intervention in that process will result in a specific outcome. Some interventions may suppress the repair activity, while others can speed up the process. In an attempt to manage symptoms, some drugs can put stress back onto the system. Carefully managed, drugs may reduce symptoms while still allowing the process to move through to the second (repair) phase. This is, of course, the aim. In some cases, however, a course of drugs may also stress the system back into the first phase, so delaying access to the second phase of repair. Some drugs may even stop the process altogether, but they do not stop the need for the process to occur. A particularly obvious example is the use of cortisol creams to treat eczema. These creams certainly reduce the symptoms, but as soon as the creams are no longer applied, the symptoms come back, sometimes even worse than before.

It may be entirely appropriate to control fungi, mycobacteria, bacteria and viruses - especially if their presence and activity is extreme and troubling. The shift in understanding that I am sharing with you is that fungi, bacteria and viruses did not *cause* the problem; instead, they are engaged in the process of repairing a problem that needs to be addressed at its root cause. The two-phase process needs to be undergone and completed in order to return to health and, most importantly, the original trigger and trauma needs to be dealt with and released if the disease is to be completely healed.

Just imagine how useful this information about the two phases can be, when working with your GP to encourage the body to move through the healing process. If you know what your medical or pharmaceutical intervention will do, you can deploy it much more effectively to move *through* the process, rather than to hold yourself within it.

Getting stuck in the process

This model of the two phases is the most basic and simple description of a dis-ease process with no complications, but as we know, life is not like that. An individual's view of the world can be extremely complicated and may lead to complex patterns of response. Nonetheless, by using this simple model we can make sense of more complex dis-ease processes and symptom patterns by helping to define which phase we may be stuck in and working backwards to the original triggers and traumatic events.

Getting stuck in the first phase

It is possible to experience a traumatic event and to become locked in the stress phase of that trauma. This can happen if there is no resolution or if the danger remains present or impending. It might also happen that there is a brief resolution, but that the trigger is reactivated very soon after, and to a greater degree than, the resolution. This means that any repair that was begun is halted by a greater degree of stress being placed back on the tissue. Let's use our four examples from this chapter to examine what might happen under these circumstances.

- **Brainstem, first phase increase of cells in the tonsils**

  Stress trigger - If nine-year-old Chloe repeatedly experiences her friends having treats that she is not allowed and her parents did not keep their promise of strawberries as an attractive alternative, or if Chloe decided that she still wanted what her friends were having despite her mother's promise of an alternative treat, Chloe would experience a re-triggering of the trauma – having a 'taste', but having it taken away. Chloe's tonsils would be sent the message to increase cells in response to each of the triggers, and would become enlarged. Unless this issue is resolved, Chloe would remain stuck in the first phase.

  Other brainstem-associated tissues that continue to increase cell production in the stress phase include: lung alveoli, liver parenchyma, the pancreas, small and large intestine, uterus, fallopian tube and prostate.

- **Cerebellum, first phase increase of cells in mammary (breast) tissue**

  Stress trigger - In the case of Emma, if the worry and threat of argument is ongoing, the cells of her breast tissue will continue to increase, eventually creating a tumour in the breast. Without a resolution of the situation, there will be no decrease of cells - only an increase, which might be diagnosed as a benign fibroadenoma (solid lump) or a lobular breast cancer.

Other cerebellum-associated tissues that continue to increase cell production in the stress phase include: pericardium (membrane around the heart), pleura (membranes around the lungs), meninges (membranes protecting the brain and central nervous system) and dermis of the skin.

- **Cerebral medulla, first phase decrease of cells in the knee-joint tissue**

Stress trigger - Eric did not feel able to progress in his work, because he felt unable to compete with younger men who also do what he does, so the tissue in his knee joints began to degrade and become thinner. Remember that in the case of the cerebral medulla, both phases must be completed for the bio-logical purpose to be fulfilled and the tissue to be completely healed and stronger than before. So, being stuck in this first phase with no resolution will mean that Eric will continue to experience a continued weakening of his knee joints and possibly of the supporting tendons and ligaments. There will be no pain in the stress phase, because pain is the result of the repair activity. However, the increased weakness in his joints will mean that they become very easily damaged.

Other cerebral medulla-associated tissues that continue to decrease cell production in the stress phase include: tendons, ligaments, muscles, bones, lymph glands, kidney parenchyma, the adrenal cortex, ovaries and testicles.

- **Cerebral cortex, first phase decrease of cells in the epidermis of the skin**

Stress trigger - Alice wanted contact with her brother and her family, but could not touch or hold onto him. For Alice, this situation remained in stress for a long time. Each time she re-lived the hurt of the separation and loss of contact, she re-triggered the stress

85

phase, bringing about a further decrease in her epidermal tissue and desensitising of her skin. Alice noticed that her hands were very pale, cold and dry and that she was unable to feel things. There was no sensitivity, especially in her fingertips or in the heels of her hands. She was stuck in the stress phase by continual re-triggering of her separation conflict.

Other cerebral cortex-associated tissues that continue to decrease cells in the stress phase include: larynx muscle and mucous membrane (mucosa), coronary veins and arteries, bladder inner mucous membrane (mucosa), teeth enamel, alpha and beta islet cells of the pancreas[28], bronchial muscle and mucous membranes, small curvature of the stomach, retinas, liver bile and pancreatic duct mucous membranes (mucosa) and gall bladder.

In each of these case studies, it is possible to see how becoming stuck in the stress phase can create symptoms. We are able to see how the tissue responds according to its nature and function in an attempt to resolve the situation and to bring relief to the original emotional trauma.

Although there was not an immediate danger or a direct threat to survival, each case study demonstrates how we interpret the world around us predominantly in terms of how we can survive and function. We are a complex array of thoughts, beliefs and perceptions as well as tissues and organs, functioning together as one.

In each of the case studies, there was a strong perception that something was fundamentally wrong and that the person must adapt to cope in order to survive. We all have such beliefs hard-wired into our subconsciouses and it is with these survival rules that we interpret the world.

---

28 The pancreas contains different areas of hormone-secreting tissue, called the islets of Langerhans, which have four types of cells. Alpha cells produce glucogen and beta cells release insulin; both hormones are crucial to various metabolic processes

Getting stuck in the second phase - Many of the diseases that we know more commonly are actually symptoms stuck in the second phase. These include aches and pains of the musculo-skeletal system, coughs, colds, fevers and flu. We become stuck in this second phase when we have experienced a resolution to the original trauma or re-triggered event, so that we spend most of our time in regeneration, but with momentary dips back into stress when we revisit the problem either literally or in our minds. We do not spend long in the stress phase and we are able to resolve the issue quickly each time, but by constantly revisiting the trigger event we do not allow the healing phase to complete and to return us to full health. Instead, a loop may be created in which the resulting symptoms re-trigger the original stressor.

Let's examine the same case studies with possible symptoms in the second phase.

- **Brainstem, second phase decrease of cells in the tonsils**

  Regeneration trigger, second phase - If Chloe were to be reminded of her friends eating their ice cream and it still upset her, even though she could quickly reconcile the issue with her reward of strawberries, she would briefly re-trigger the stress phase and not complete the second phase of regeneration, in which the excess cells are broken down by mycobacteria. This re-triggering would send the message to make more tissue again. If Chloe were once more reminded that she has her strawberries instead and quickly felt better again, she would go back into the second (regeneration) phase. This constant, brief re-triggering followed by resolution, even if only by her thoughts, would be enough to hold Chloe in the second phase and to stop her from going beyond it back into full health.

87

- **Cerebellum, second phase decrease of cells in mammary (breast) tissue**

  Regeneration trigger, second phase - If Emma had not elected to go for surgery for her mammary tumour, she would have experienced either an encapsulation of the nodes or a degradation of the nodes by *Mycobacterium tuberculosis*. If the issue had been resolved, but Emma was still re-triggered by the fear that further arguments could happen, she would swing between the first and second phases and the mycobacterial function would increase in the second phase.

  In this case, it is important to realise that, although Emma opted for surgery, it would still be beneficial to work on her original problem of fear or worry about argument in the nest. Releasing the root cause would still allow the best possible healing for Emma and would help to ensure that there would not be a re-growth of the tumour.

- **Cerebral medulla, second phase increase of cells in the knee-joint tissue**

  Regeneration trigger, second phase - In this programme, we see how strength is built up in the tissue during the second phase. After the initial decrease in cells, the tissue of tendons, ligaments, joints, muscles, and bones all regenerate to become stronger by the end of the second phase. However, this is when pain is experienced. Similarly, a bodybuilder who goes to the gym to build up his muscles must rest after his workout to allow repair to take place. This is when he feels swelling, stiffness and pain. It is during this repair phase that Eric could easily be reminded of his original conflict about not being able to compete with younger men. In fact, the pain we experience in the regeneration phase of the musculo-skeletal system is frequently perceived as a failure of the body and is often age-related. So, if Eric resolves his issue and feels better about himself, but then goes into repair and gets pain in his knees, he could easily trigger himself back into the stress phase by this very pattern of thought. When he feels better again, he will once more enter into repair, but this will also be when the tissue swells and becomes painful while it is regenerating.

So if Eric doesn't realise that his pain is actually a sign of healing, he will get anxious about it and might well send himself back into the first phase again. This can become a vicious circle, leading to degenerative joint and muscle problems, as is evident in arthritis.

So, I hope it is clear that an awareness of the dis-ease process makes all the difference! Understanding that each of my illnesses was a process in which I had allowed myself to become trapped, changed the way I viewed my illnesses and myself. Knowing that something could be done to create movement through that process gave me power to take small steps to begin my full recovery. I understood my bad back much better and began to pay attention to when it hurt, or when the pain eased off. I began to have a dialogue with my body.

- **Cerebral cortex, second phase increase of cells in the epidermis of the skin**

Regeneration trigger, second phase - Once Alice had released some of the emotion concerning missing her family and contact with her brother, she was able to enter into the second phase, when her skin could begin to regenerate. The symptoms of eczema – red, dry, hot, flaky skin, itching, cracking and soreness – are all present due to the skin being under repair. Because contact is such a deep issue, the eczema can become a stress trigger in itself. A person often feels that with these symptoms they are not going to be able to touch the person or thing that they want to touch. If they return into the stress phase because of this pattern of thought, the symptoms will disappear again and they may briefly feel better about their situation as they show fewer symptoms. If the original emotional issue is still not dealt with, however, they will swing between being stressed, finding some degree of resolution by coming to terms with the lack of contact, and then being re-triggered by the physical symptoms in the regeneration phase.

The healing peak

If we examine the diagram of the two phases (See *Nature's two phases* of disease earlier in this chapter), we can see that there is a peak halfway through the second phase. We call this the 'healing peak' or 'healing crisis' - I think 'crisis' sounds a bit frightening, so I prefer to use the term 'peak'. This is a very important stage of the healing phase, because it is critical in moving the healing part of the process from the first element, when the swelling and activity are at their highest, to the second element, when the tissue begins to normalise and return to its original state and function. In the first element of the second phase, we experience the most intense repair with activity of fungi, mycobacteria and viruses, before reaching the healing peak.

> ❝❝ *By recognising what the symptoms represent, we will be able to decode the information and analyse the root cause of the dis-ease.* ❞

The healing peak serves a number of functions. At the peak, the water that has swollen the organ tissue is expelled and there is a shift to remove the degraded tissue. This is often seen in the form of a phlegmy cough or a runny nose, for example. In the case of muscles, there may be cramps and in nerve repair there may be a firing of the nerves.

This point in the repair is critical, especially in such repairs as, for example, the myocardium (muscular tissue) of the heart. Triggered by feelings of being overwhelmed, the myocardium weakens in the stress phase, then swells with water and repairs in the regeneration phase. It is important to be aware that during the healing peak of the repair phase, a heart attack could occur when the muscle of the heart goes into spasm. So, in META-Health we maintain an awareness of where the client is in the process and examine all the contributing factors, to create the best and safest scenario to move through this critical part of the process. Understanding the process forewarns us and we have clear guidelines regarding severity, timing and symptoms. All of this information is vital to avoid complications and any danger of reaching a critical threshold. This information allows us to plan what steps to take in controlling the safest passage through the healing.

The organ-brain-psyche connection

So far we have mostly examined tissue response to the trigger, but all the time that this is happening, the psyche and brain are responding also. Whenever there is a dip back into the stress phase, there is a psychological shift back into obsessive thinking about the problem. This also happens when the healing peak occurs, because there is a dip back to the original issue, in order to test for completion. At this point, there is a risk of being re-triggered back into the stress phase.

When repair occurs in the organ, water also goes to the corresponding relay in the brain to assist in the repair of the relay. This water in the relay can also cause a headache by increasing pressure on the brain in the skull. This is different to other types of headaches caused by specific triggers.

Real or perceived threats

When a person triggers a bio-logical response, the threat does not have to be actual. There does not need to be a real threat to survival - such as a hungry tiger in front of you - for triggering to occur. Most often we are our own worst enemies, by not letting go of past issues. We replay things over and over in our minds and build bigger and more complicated stories around them, so that they come to represent far more than was originally the case.

We connect beliefs and build complex belief systems that are designed to keep us safe, but may actually end up triggering our bodies into compensatory behaviour on our behalf.

We have explored the main principles of META-Health and looked at how the body-mind works together. This now gives us a foundation to be able to decipher some of the messages from our body. By recognising what the symptoms represent, we will be able to decode the information and analyse the root cause of the dis-ease.

At this stage, I think it is a good idea to ask yourself which symptoms you would like to understand. What underlying truth about your health are you curious to reveal? What breakthrough would you like to have in your life that would help you to move forwards?

The answers are all there. Your body has been trying to tell you.

5. De-coding the META messages

"Your body is an absolute mirror of your mind. As you worry, your body shows it. As you love, your body shows it. As you are overwhelmed, your body shows it. As you are angry, your body shows it. Every cell of your body is being allowed or resisted by the way you feel. 'My physical state is a direct reflection of how I feel', instead of 'How I feel is a direct reflection of my physical state'. **Abraham/Esther Hicks**[29]

In order to make the connection between the symptoms of dis-ease and your emotions, you need to understand what is happening in the tissue of the organ. When you understand the purpose of the tissue adaptation, you can identify the type of conflict that is at the root cause of the problem. The trigger could be a traumatic event, a thought or the memory of an event; it could even be an inherited perception of certain types of event. By releasing the energy and trapped emotions from the trauma it is possible to bring about a change in perspective. When a trauma is released and learning occurs, there can be an almost instant change in the body. I see this time and time again with clients - as they evolve their energy states, their bodies respond with changing symptoms.

When working with certain types of dis-ease, such as aches and pains or skin issue, it is possible to test whether you have found the right triggers by re-associating with the emotion of the original event. When you re-associate with the stress of the event, the symptoms will ease. When you re-associate with the resolution of that event, the symptoms will come back if you have entered into the rest and repair phase.

---

29 *The Law of Attraction - How to Make It Work for You*, Esther and Jerry Hicks (The Teachings of Abraham), Hay House Inc, Carlsbad, CA, USA, 2006

It is very useful to use this simple association technique to demonstrate the power that you have to turn your symptoms on and off with your thoughts. The important thing is for you to understand that your body responds directly to what you think and when symptoms occur in the second phase, your body is actually healing itself and not breaking down. This means that you can support your body through the healing process and out the other side, instead of re-triggering the stress and having to repeat the process over and over again, with the risk of creating long-term dis-ease.

There are several factors that need to be taken into consideration when analysing the root cause of a specific dis-ease. And, let's be clear here, I do not claim to be making a medical diagnosis. In META-Health practice, an investigation is undertaken into the emotional root cause analysis of a medical condition that has already been diagnosed by a qualified medical doctor - unless the META-Health coach or practitioner is also a qualified doctor, in which case she/he would use her/his skills in combination.

If clients come with a self-diagnosed condition or symptom, it is far more difficult to pinpoint the root cause. Without a correct medical diagnosis, it is not always possible to define the actual tissue involved and therefore the associated brain layer, theme and underlying traumatic event. For example, I worked with a lady who has an irritating skin condition, but had not had a medical diagnosis, because she was too embarrassed to show her symptoms to the doctor. We discussed the symptoms and in particular the timings of when they began, when they appeared to disappear and when they got worse. However, without a medical diagnosis, we did not know if the problem was originating in the dermis or epidermis of the skin, which would suggest two very different lines of enquiry. If the problem were generated in the dermis, for example, there would be different symptoms in the stress and regeneration phases – with an increase of cells in the stress phase, followed by a decrease of cells in the regeneration phase (typical of acne). Conversely, if the problem were to be medically diagnosed as arising in the epidermis, there would be a reduction of cells in the stress phase, followed by an increase of cells in the regeneration phase (as in eczema). So, information about symptoms does not mean much without the vital information derived from a proper medical diagnosis.

In the absence of this information, it was necessary to discuss the themes of both the dermis and epidermis with this client, to see which resonated most with her emotional state around the symptoms.

- Dermis > cerebellum > theme: protection and integrity.
- Epidermis > cerebral cortex > theme: contact, territorial, social.

I asked her questions about the problem' and explored the different aspects of the two themes. When I asked about contact in the affected area and what this area represented to her, there was not much response, but when I asked what protection and integrity meant to her in this area, she immediately became emotional.

It is possible to work in this way with a client, but I must reiterate that, even if a traumatic event is identified and the symptoms change as a result of working on that event and the perceptions and beliefs associated with it, it still cannot be considered a medical diagnosis.

The META-Health analysis

The purpose of a META-Health analysis is to empower you to explore the relationship between your symptoms and traumatic, stressful events you have experienced as well as your underlying thoughts and feelings. It is vital that you make your own connections, so the investigation is designed to collect the relevant information to formulate a specific question. That question should enable you to know where to look for the link, to pinpoint the causal event or trigger. You need to know that you are shining a light in the right place to discover the right event. As you follow the steps (below) in the investigation, you might like to think about an illness of your own, or perhaps of someone you know.

I recently did a demonstration with a participant in a META-Health Introductory Training session. Amy[30] is a gifted therapist and offered to take part in the

---

30 Thank you to Amy Branton, EFT & Matrix Practitioner (www. freehearteft.co.uk) for kindly giving permission for this personal information to be used in this book and on the training video of that session.

demonstration since she had a pain in her heel that she did not understand (for a video of this training demo, see www.intoalignment.com).

We will use Amy's example to demonstrate META-Health diagnostic questioning techniques. So, what do we need to know to make a META-Health analysis?

- **The complaint** *What is your complaint and what are the symptoms?*

Amy complained of a pain beneath her left heel when she moved forwards, possibly a tendon, muscle or bone.

- **Location** *What is the position and purpose of the organ tissue? What does it do?*

Although we cannot define which part of the heel is affected without a doctor's diagnosis, we do know that the heel is part of the musculo-skeletal system. It was important to get Amy to move around a little to find out what specific movement made the heel hurt, because this tells us which action is relevant to the situation.

Amy's heel hurt when she stood with her weight on it and, in particular, when she stepped forwards.

- **Dominance** *Which is your dominant side?*

We know that Amy's left heel hurts, so we need to determine what relevance the left side has to Amy's emotions. We can focus our attention further by testing which is Amy's dominant side. We do this by asking Amy to clap a few times and then to relax and seeing which hand is uppermost. A good indication is to observe which thumb is on top.

The body responds to our perception of the world by processing things and people that we regard as equal to us - such as our careers, partners, friends, colleagues or siblings - on our dominant side. The body expresses what we perceive to be in a nurturing position for us - such as our homes, parents or children - on our non-dominant side. (My parents because they nurture me; my children because I nurture them.) This perception is very subjective. For example, one person may see their pet dog as their best friend, which would show on that person's dominant side, whereas another person might perceive their dog as their baby - as do I with my little Yorkie, Fern. This perception can change in a given context, so whereas I see my brother as my equal in some situations, I may see him in a nurturing role when I am taking care of him in another.

Amy's left hand was uppermost when she clapped, so this tells us that she is left-hand dominant. This is not the same as knowing which hand Amy writes with, because this can be simply the result of learned behaviour. Once we have this information, we can conclude that a problem with Amy's left heel is regarding an issue associated with her career or an equal person or partner.

- **Organ tissue** *What is the specific organ tissue and associated brain layer?*

We know that the musculo-skeletal system – tendons, ligaments, muscles, bones – are all formed from the new mesoderm germ layer, associated with the cerebral medulla.

- **Theme and conflict** *What is the theme of the brain layer and the specific organ-tissue conflict?*

Cerebral Medulla > issues of movement and strength and self worth.

'I am not good enough or strong enough to do something ...'

Left heel > Standing, moving forwards, onwards, upwards.

- **Adaptation** *What change does this tissue make in the stress phase (cell increase or cell decrease)?*

In the stress phase (sympathetic nervous system), we see a cell decrease. The bio-logical purpose for this programme is to enter the second phase in order to repair even stronger than before.

- **Timing** *When did the symptoms start? Is there a time when they are worse, better? Has there been a break in the symptoms?*

Amy remembers the symptoms were there a few months ago, but this last time they have been present for about eight weeks.

- **Phases** *Where in the two phases are you? Confirm with other symptoms: hot or cold, active or sleepy, obsessive or supine?*

Because Amy is in pain, we know that she is in the second phase - in regeneration. This is when the organ swells with water while the tissue is repairing. Amy has been in this second phase for about eight weeks.

- **Posing the question** *Formulate the question that will assist the client in locating the traumatic event or thought that triggered the process.*

We have ascertained the following information:

- Left heel means not good enough or strong enough to move forwards in a career or equal relationship.
- Approximately eight weeks in second phase.
- Therefore, some eight weeks ago there was a turning point (a 'resolution') when something happened that made Amy feel *better* about the situation. This caused her to shift from the stress phase into the regeneration phase.
- The 'something' that caused this shift will be the emotional trigger we are looking for, to help Amy resolve her underlying issue.

I asked Amy what had happened about eight weeks ago, just before the pain in her heel started. Had she, for example, felt *better* about something relating to her career or an equal person, with regard to which she had not previously been able to move forwards?

Amy immediately realised what had happened. She had begun to get her first clients in her new business and realised that everything was going to be fine and that she could be successful.

Prior to the resolution turning point, Amy had been in a period of stress and self-doubt. In the basic model of the two phases of illness, there is an equal balance of time and intensity between the stress phase and the regeneration phase. This means that, if Amy had been emerging from the regeneration phase after eight weeks, we would look first to the shift trigger event when she entered that phase (eight weeks before), and then to a further eight weeks before that, when we could have looked for the UDIN moment that had caused her to enter the stress phase. In this case, however, Amy had become stuck in the second phase by re-triggering her thoughts about failure and this had prevented her from completing the healing process. This re-triggering was because the underlying issue was based on a number of beliefs about Amy's self-worth. Amy was now able to focus on these issues and to resolve them as a result of the META-Health analysis.

- **Status** - *What is the status of the process? Is the status stuck in first phase, second phase, re-triggered or re-occurring?*

  Amy had been re-triggering the process and had become stuck in the second phase. She was in regeneration for a period of time, but kept making quick references back to the stressor. There was a fear that she would not be able to sustain the new work, accompanied by a fear of things that had happened in the past being repeated.

- *What is the META message (belief or core belief)?*

The message from the body was telling Amy that she did not feel strong enough or good enough to move forwards in her career. Amy was able to see how her beliefs about her ability were affecting her outlook and her health. It has also brought to light the fear she was holding about the past, which she had not realised was affecting her so much.

> **" Since I learned META-Health and energy therapy I have been able to change my life and my physical, mental and emotional state. Things still trigger me, but they are signs and messages for me now. I thank them and I follow them to discover something about myself that I need to understand. "**

The message from Amy's body -that she did not feel strong or good enough to move forwards in her career - stemmed from a previous experience of setting up a business, which had not been as successful as she had wanted. The belief she formed at that time had been: 'I'm a failure.' As a high achiever who was used to being successful in her career, this belief was one of the main catalysts that eventually led to depression and a breakdown. So embarking on a new business venture a few years later had triggered her fear of another failure (stress phase).

If she had perceived her first business venture as a valuable experience from which she had learned a lot, rather than viewing it - and herself - as a total failure, Amy could have created a positive belief about herself that would have helped her to move forwards, rather than feeling fearful about trying again. This is an example of the power that our beliefs can hold over us.

Amy's ability to connect her physical issue with a specific event and set of beliefs has meant that she could resolve the emotional issue by changing the belief that was affecting her health. We will briefly explore some change techniques later in this book.

For more complex issues, we use a range of tools to help the client tune into the information and bring the memories to the surface. I often use EFT slow tapping, which is a technique of tapping slowly on one of the meridian acupressure points while concentrating on the problem. It is surprising what information comes up.

Using the META-Health information and questioning techniques, we can unscramble complex health issues and build a clear picture of someone's symptoms and illness. We can form a picture of the physical, psychological and emotional terrain of someone's life. What starts as a series of simple questions takes us back into the deep workings of the mind and the way that each of us makes sense of ourselves and of the world in which we live. If we can learn to read the signs and listen to the messages, we might find that our bodies and minds are communicating as one all the time. Things could be quite different if you were fully aware of your thoughts and beliefs.

Since I learned META-Health and energy therapy I have been able to change my life and my physical, mental and emotional state. Things still trigger me, but they are signs and messages for me now. I thank them and I follow them to discover something about myself that I need to understand. I had a great childhood, but we all have our misperceptions and form beliefs and decisions that shape our paths through life. I have learned more about myself and my life in the last few years than I ever dreamed I could. My life really did begin at forty!

What message was my back telling me?

I suffered with a bad back for years. It seemed as though I had some form of lumbar pain most of the time. Sometimes I could barely walk because the nerve down into my right leg would ache so much. I didn't sleep well and, if I exercised, it would be even worse afterwards. I labelled myself as someone with 'a bad back' and began to identify with that label.

It was not until I discovered META-Health that I was able to understand what my back was telling me. Amazing, really: from understanding that specific aspect of my health, I was able to connect it to my other beliefs and thoughts and piece together a whole network of physical and psychological symptoms. It was even possible to understand my depression and aggressive outbursts and ultimately the drink and drug addictions that I had used as coping mechanisms.

Seeking resolution and evolution

It may seem hard to believe that damaging and destructive behaviour could be a way of seeking resolution and peace. My own behaviour certainly did not approach anything like peace. When I was at my lowest, I felt utterly helpless and frustrated at the world and my situation and found it impossible to manage my emotions. My lower-back pain was only part of my problems at that time, but it is interesting to see now how my back was an indicator of what was going on beneath the surface of my life, although I wasn't consciously aware of it.

As we have discussed, all musculo-skeletal problems - that is, bones, muscles, tendons, ligaments and joints - are associated to the cerebral medulla brain layer. The cerebral medulla responds first with a decrease of cells in the stress phase, followed by an increase of cells in the regeneration phase. The full process must be completed for the bio-logical programme to have served its purpose – that is, to reinforce the tissue to be stronger next time.

Imagine a bodybuilder working out at the gym. During his weight-lifting session, he will lift more than he is comfortably able to, with a clear intention of fatiguing and damaging his muscles. This is the stress phase. It is important that he then rest this set of muscles, so that they can repair in order to grow stronger than before. During the repair of the muscle, tissue swelling and oedema (fluid build-up) can cause pain and cramp until the muscle finally starts to return to normal. It will be stronger than before and better able to cope the next time it is called upon to lift heavy weights. When the bodybuilder returns to the gym, he will be able to lift the same weight more easily. If he wants to build more muscle, he will again deliberately damage it by lifting heavier weights and repeat the process to maintain an increase in muscle.

Physical issues of the musculo-skeletal system are about not being strong enough or good enough to be able to do something. In the same way, the bodybuilder sends the message to his muscle 'I am not strong enough to lift this weight' so that a signal is sent to the muscle to go through a process of breakdown, followed by strengthening and repair. The muscle will then be strong enough to cope with increased demands.

Each part of the human body has a dedicated function, and each bone, muscle and joint does something specific: our heads think; our necks hold our heads up; our shoulders carry things; our thoracic spines hold us upright with shoulders back; our arms hold onto or push things away; our hands grip; our ribs protect our organs; our pelvises hold our sexuality; our hips hold our positions and stand our ground; our legs move us forwards; our knees allow us to flex and change direction; our ankles and feet propel us onwards and upwards.

The spine is our core column. At its base is the coccyx and the sacrum, which is part of the pelvis; next are the lumbar vertebrae. The lumbar region supports the rest of the back from the base and enables you to 'stand by yourself'. It is the part of the body that links you standing up and standing tall; it represents you being yourself and either supporting yourself or being accepted by others.

My personal back problems affected the muscles and nerves in my lumbar region. Some days were worse than others and when it was excruciating I used painkillers. There was no discernible pattern to the pain, until I discovered META-Health.

When I felt people did not understand me (which was most of my life since childhood), I felt that I could not be myself. People didn't, or couldn't, accept me if they didn't understand me. I had a fear of being misunderstood or misjudged. Clearly, I still have not fully resolved this issue, because I am getting a pain in my lower right back and down the back of my right leg as I type this. Why would that be? Why would it hurt now?

If you remember the bodybuilder, when the stress phase is over, the body can enter into the second phase of rest and repair, and it is then that the pain starts. By writing about this belief, I feel I am making myself understood, so I enter into the repair phase. It is interesting that I didn't know I was under any degree of stress in this regard. My underlying belief that 'I am not understood' lies so deep and sits so quietly in the subconscious that I expect that belief to be true in every instant of my life without questioning it. Most of the time I do not notice it is there and I have done a great deal of work on it. My back is now my barometer for this belief. My body reminds me of what I am thinking and to what degree I am thinking it.

Remember, with the musculo-skeletal system there is no pain during the first phase, in stress. The pain comes in the second phase once the issue has been resolved, either practically or mentally and emotionally. When the problem is solved, the trigger is no longer active and I enter into the second phase - the repair. This is when the swelling and pain occur. So, to have a 'bad back', you must feel *better* about the issue that previously had made you feel that you were not strong enough.

Learning the lesson

I no longer get a crippling backache, but I do get the odd twinge on the right side and sometimes discomfort in the right sciatic nerve. Because the connection between the belief and the back pain is so specific, I am able to focus on my personal perceptions to investigate my thought patterns. There is a quick-fire chain of thought that follows from a trigger straight to the end result. In this case, if my back hurts, it means I feel better because you understand me. My chain of thought is: now you validated me; now you understood me; now I am supported; now I can support myself; now I can be myself. The location of this pain is relative to how this belief personally impacts me. However, for someone else their sense of not being validated might mean to them that they are dirty, or they are unloved. In that case, a different biological response would occur. I felt I could not stand up and be myself, that I would not be understood.

> " We see the world through the filters that we created when we were younger and our world, in turn, is created by these filters. "

It took some time to work out this chain of thought because it had previously been completely subconscious. I now know that my triggers are specific to people who are close to me and specifically with regard to understanding my morals or intentions. This is the connection between 'being strong enough to be myself' and 'not being understood'. For example, a specific negative thought would be: 'I would never do that. How could you think that of me!' The belief would be: 'When I am myself, you don't understand me ... whatever I do, you will still think badly of me...I can't be me; I can't make you understand.'

Finding the gift

If you had said to me a few years ago that my bad back was a gift, well, let's just say I would not have agreed! So much else in my life was in a mess, due to this belief system and a few others, that I saw my bad back as just another part of the problem.

The way we view the world is the way we act in the world. If we believe that people will judge us, we will be ever ready to face their judgments. If we feel that people will think we are stupid, we will go through life prepared to be treated as if we are stupid. And if nobody treats us like that we will probably go out of our way to act stupid so that they do! We see the world through the filters that we created when we were younger and our world, in turn, is created by these filters.

I felt misunderstood as a child and have grown up believing that people would not understand or believe me when I talk about my feelings or myself. In turn, this made it increasingly difficult for me to be myself. I felt I was not strong enough to be myself – this belief meant I could be triggered with the lower back problem. If you met me, this would not be particularly apparent, since I have also spent my life learning ways to compensate, to explain myself well. However, the belief still lay underneath and to some extent still lingers, in particular with reference to being believed about my moral intentions.

Now that I know this, I can work on my perceptions and the limiting beliefs that affect the way I see the world. Using such energy therapies as EFT and Matrix Reimprinting[31], I have visited the relevant memories and released the stuck emotion and energy regarding negative beliefs. The transformation of

---

31 See www.matrixreimprinting.com for more information; also *Matrix Reimprinting Using EFT*(Karl Dawson & Sacha Allenby, Hay House UK Ltd, London, 2010) and *Emotional Freedom Techniques for Dummies* (Helena Fone, John Wiley & Sons Ltd, Chichester, UK, 2008).

these beliefs has made such a change in my life. I am who I am; I am doing what I love.

There is an important distinction between changing the world around you and changing your view of the world. One way to resolve an issue is to change the things around you. To deal with my problem I could have learned to communicate more clearly - which in fact I did. I studied graphics, to communicate through drawings, and trained to be a teacher and learned to deliver complex ideas in a simple and clear way. I now receive regular compliments for my clarity, which of course has been a great help in my training sessions and seminars. However, it did not really solve my problem, which was that I expected those close to me to misunderstand or misjudge me. No matter how well things went, or how closely people paid attention or listened, I was ready for that one moment when I felt I 'knew' that they were judging me wrongly. I was waiting to be upset.

By evolving the e-motion that was stuck around early memories, I was able to take a different perspective. As a general rule, I do not have the belief that people will not understand or believe me or my intentions, but on occasion there are still triggers around this issue. This means that there is still a little more work to be done.

Attracting what you need, not what you want

When we have a lesson to learn in life, we are given every opportunity to get the message. We will keep attracting the same lesson until we finally understand what we need to know. Have you ever asked yourself why you always end up in the same kind of relationship, for example? What is it about yourself that you didn't learn or accept yet? Can you transform your perceptions and stop attracting the same lessons?

It appeared to me that I was misunderstood. I found at work and in my relationships that this would always end up being the case. Not all the time, but it seemed that way whenever it really mattered to me. I learned to watch out for it, to be ready to respond and I was always right, of course! I expected to be misjudged and so, to protect myself, I would judge other people's ability to judge me. I was always trying to work out everything I might need to know so as not to be misjudged. Quite exhausting, really! It takes a lot of energy to remain so vigilant, especially if you are constantly preparing to defend your corner or make your point.

It takes a big leap to move from the position of 'bad things happen to me' to that of 'I am doing this to myself' and it was not until my life fell apart that I was ready to make the necessary changes to turn things around. It was then that I was able to listen and learn.

I think, therefore I am

I didn't think there was a problem with my beliefs. They weren't even beliefs to me - they were simply 'the TRUTH'! Our beliefs are so true for us that we do not see outside them. We do not see them as simply beliefs. Have you ever considered that the way you look at the world is just a construction of your beliefs? That what you hold as absolutely true is only true as you see it?

Let us look at some beliefs and see how the body's response to a particular trigger might be related to a belief. For example, someone who has a trauma in which they are unable to define a limit or a position or to mark her/his territory, will trigger a response in the bladder inner lining or mucous membrane (mucosa). Have you noticed how animals urinate to mark their territories? The bladder mucosa is a tissue associated with the cerebral cortex and so we know that there is a reduction of cells in the stress phase, during which there will be a thinning of the lining of the bladder. This makes the bladder bigger so it can hold more urine - the better to mark our territory or position, just as animals do.

Cannot mark territory > cerebral cortex > bladder mucosa

There is the initial perception 'I cannot define my position or territory' and underlying that will be a further thought, or chain of thought, for example:

107

- I cannot say 'no' to people.
- If I say 'no' to people, I will be a bad person.
- If I am a bad person, no one will like me.
- If no one likes me and rejects me, I will be alone.

These are not the kinds of belief that we wear on the surface. They are buried deep down and yet are fundamental to the formation of our day-to-day lives. Consider each of the following beliefs and rate how true that statement is for you out of 100 per cent (0 per cent being 'this is not at all true for me' and 100 per cent being 'this it completely true for me'). Be honest and answer quickly by tuning into your gut feeling, rather than trying to work out the answer consciously.

- I am unlovable
- I have to change to be loved
- I am ugly
- I am alone
- I am a bad person
- People take advantage of me
- People misunderstand me
- The world is a dangerous place
- Bad things happen to me
- I can't cope
- I can't do it
- There is not enough
- I will never do better
- I make bad decisions
- I am not good enough
- It is different for me
- I will never be happy
- I will never be healthy
- People leave me

- People let me down
- It's all my fault
- I have to make things right
- Everything is hard work

In energy therapy, we consider these to be 'core beliefs' that permeate many different areas of our life. Someone who has the core belief 'I will never be happy' would see evidence of this in their family, their work and their relationships and would believe it to be evidentially true.

How did you do? The aim of course is to have 0 per cent, but I have never known that to be the case for anyone. I encourage you to review your results with a curious mind and perhaps to be open to witnessing where those beliefs may be affecting your life-view.

Imagine your beliefs as 'rose-tinted glasses' - only these are more like having glasses with dark and dirty lenses. When we see a person or the world through rose-tinted glasses, we see them as wonderful and faultless - the negative aspects are filtered out. When we wear the glasses of our beliefs, we filter out the more positive aspects and only see the negative things that we expect to see. With your 'the world is a dangerous place' glasses on, the world really is dangerous to you. You are sure to find danger if you seek it out in everything and filter out the rest.

Forming beliefs

By the time you are seven, you have already formed your core beliefs and are using them to make sense of the world. So where did they come from? Look back at the beliefs list again and answer the same questions on behalf of one of your parents. Do you notice any similarities? We either inherit our beliefs from our parents or primary carers, or we acquire them during events of our formative years.

Our beliefs are not necessarily formed from major traumas in our lives. We form beliefs and decisions from simple situations that we may have misinterpreted. It is even possible for a baby to make a decision or belief in the womb. A mother who is stressed and upset transmits the same chemical responses to those emotions to the baby. The baby therefore 'experiences' those emotions. Before it is even born, the baby has learned stress and, when it enters the world, it is hard-wired to identify stressful events. For some babies the belief is already formed before birth that 'the world is a dangerous place' or 'bad things will happen'.

> *Our beliefs are not necessarily formed from major traumas in our lives. We form beliefs and decisions from simple situations that we may have misinterpreted.*"

It is often the simple and innocuous events that go seemingly unnoticed, but that create beliefs which permeate our lives. If we come back to my own example of not being understood, I used Matrix Reimprinting to revisit a clear memory, in order to identify when and where it had occurred. It took me back to the age of four.

All it takes to create a trauma is helplessness and a threat to survival. Imagine how the world looks to a child of four. It is easy for such a child to interpret a dismissive response from a harassed mother as a rejection and a threat to survival.

When we have a traumatic experience, we create amnesia around it in order to deaden our conscious memory of the pain. However, all the information that was around at the time of our trauma is recorded subconsciously, so that we can make sense of the world and so that we are prepared next time a similar event occurs.

David and the colouring book

When I was five I loved colouring books. Every Christmas I would have a new colouring book, with a big pack of felt-tip pens. I would work my way through the book, picking my favourite pictures to colour in, until the book was full. I particularly loved doing it because my mum would occasionally colour one in too and I loved to see her engrossed in a quiet moment for herself, colouring in my book. I was always praised for being so neat and for not going over the lines.

For a while, my mum looked after her friend's little boy, David. Because his mum didn't finish work until after we came from playschool, David would come home with us to play until his mum arrived.

I have always had a conscious memory of David at our house one afternoon with my colouring book. David's mum was a teacher and he was imitating her, going through my book putting ticks and marks out of ten on each page. I remember being so frustrated with him ruining my book that I went up to him and kicked him in the shin. This is how I consciously remembered the event. However, when I returned to the memory properly, using Matrix Reimprinting, I realised that I had blanked out a specific part of the memory that contained the trauma preceding my violent act.

What actually had happened was that, when I saw David defacing my book, I turned to my mum in despair, pointed to David and cried, 'Mummy, stop him!' My mum, not wanting to upset the child and preferring to keep the peace, replied, 'It's all right, he's not doing any harm.' This left me totally helpless, totally isolated and frozen. I had no strategy - it was a UDIN moment. My reaction, in my helplessness and sheer frustration, was to kick him in the shin.

What is more important about that day is the beliefs that I formed as a result of what happened. I have found that there were three significant ones that were affecting my current view of the world:

111

- She does not believe me (does not believe how important the book is to me)
- She does not understand me (she does not think I should be so upset)
- I didn't do it well enough (I must do better next time for her to appreciate the importance of my feelings).

My mum didn't do anything wrong and neither did David, but the book was important to me and my feelings were not validated. I was isolated and helpless and to a four-year-old child this can feel like a threat to survival - 'no one will help me'. The beliefs I formed at this time began to create a foundation for the way that I would start to make sense of the world.

I share this story with you to demonstrate the simplicity of the event that caused such specific beliefs, leading to such repeated patterns in my life. Every client I work with has their own beliefs and patterns that go back to specific events and invariably back to core beliefs that were formed pre-six years' old.

Multiple triggers

I can connect my lower back pain to the core beliefs I formed at that time. I can also identify other dis-ease processes that were triggered at the same time - two very significant biological programmes that, when running simultaneously, caused a new behaviour to be adopted.

Two conflicts, one of 'territory anger' (my book!) and the other of 'I cannot define my position' ('you don't understand how important this is to me') struck me at the same time in this simple moment and explain the aggressive outburst that I had, kicking David in the shin. It also explains a pattern of suppressed aggression all through my frustrated teenage years and into my adulthood, especially when I felt helpless and frustrated at not being understood. We will look more at these new behaviours and at aggression in Chapter 7.

I am still a 'work in progress', as we all are. I will never, however, go back to where I was before. The depth of that despair is not possible from my current perspective. I have much work to do to release some of the energy still held in past events and I have yet to forgive myself for some of the things I have done. Yet, even when I am blindsided by an unexpected trigger, I now know that there is another way and that I have a choice. There is a reason I feel the way I do. Knowing that reason immediately gives me insight and puts me on the right track. I still have to do the work, but now I am curious about my thoughts and feelings and I take each symptom or behaviour as a signpost to give me greater insight into what I should be doing to approach greater peace and health. Recognising the META messages gives me insight into the - bio-logical - reason that I react, and therefore into the purpose of my symptoms.

Now, when I have a bad back, I am able to identify exactly what just happened to cause the pain and what my thoughts were that led me to that point. When I feel depressed, I understand exactly what my thoughts were about what someone said. When I feel a welling-up of aggression and the need to make my point and my position clear, I know what caused me to experience such a rush of emotion. Even though, in an ideal world, I would not be triggered by these things, I am for the most part present, content and healthy. I can react better in the moment and, in my own time, I can use the insight I have gained to address the changes in my health that I still need to make.

After all, the intention is not to suppress your feelings, but to allow them to process, so that you can learn and evolve, emotionally, physically, mentally and spiritually.

6. Multiple symptoms

"It is better to conquer yourself than to win a thousand battles. Then the victory is yours. It cannot be taken from you, not by angels or by demons, heaven nor hell."   **Buddha**

It would be all too easy to use the investigatory tool of META-Health and to imagine that we can simplify the complex workings of the mind and body. This is not really my aim, nor do I think it is really possible. The body and mind are divinely complex and intricate. However, if we accept the body-mind connection and are able to take responsibility for our thoughts, the body and mind become a gift and a tool of understanding.

The principles of META-Health give us an understanding of how the higher levels of our existence operate with the lower levels - the level of higher consciousness performing as a human animal. When we examine all the different diseases of the body and mind, they can be traced back to triggers that derive from fear. It seems our biological, animalistic need for survival and our spiritual need for connection are both about our continuing existence. This is the part of the puzzle that we have been missing. We are in fact divine beings having a human experience. If your experience is not a good one, what have you not understood that will enable you to change your life to have a better experience?

There is so much help and advice about stress and resilience and yet ... what's the purpose of your symptoms? What's the message? If you merely want to manage your stress and alleviate your symptoms, then, yes, you would probably encourage some healing to take place and your life would be calmer and you would be the healthier for it. But in my experience surface work alone does not calm the triggers that are in the subconscious mind. Without getting to the root cause of the problem, you are still just managing the results. META-Health gives you a deeper life message, so that not only can you release your dis-ease, but you receive a life lesson as well. To live in the

115

present moment fully and appreciatively is not to deny or forget the past. It is to accept it, to allow it and thus to let it go, taking the learning and moving on.

Unpacking complex dis-eases

Life is certainly not simple. We have many things to cope with on a day-to-day basis. We need to learn the skills of listening to our bodies, trusting our intuition and allowing our bodies and minds to work together. The fast pace of life does not really allow for this and it does take some effort to extricate oneself from old patterns and give oneself the encouragement to create new patterns.

> *Without getting to the root cause of the problem, you are still just managing the results. META-Health gives you a deeper life message, so that not only can you release your dis-ease, but you receive a life lesson as well.*"

One of the things that make it difficult to create new patterns and ways of being in the world is when we allow a label to define us. In doing so, we adopt all the energy and information that goes with that label. Illnesses have a life of their own - literally. There is a collective energy that we connect to when we assume the label of an illness and, once we start to resonate with it, we find that energy hard to shake off. We start to identify more and more with the illness as an entity in itself: '*my* depression', '*my diabetes*', '*my* fibromyalgia'.

Some illnesses named by the medical profession are a syndrome - a collection of different symptoms that have been grouped under a shared label, because they often occur together. Sometimes there is no known relationship between these symptoms, other than that they commonly appear together. This is the case for diseases such as fibromyalgia and lupus. There are variations of these illnesses based on slightly different assessment criteria. Those whose symptoms match some of the main criteria of such an illness are encouraged to assume the label of that illness.

116

Once different symptoms are grouped together as a cluster, it is almost impossible to define any one of them individually. It is easy then to accept the likelihood that you will necessarily develop the other symptoms at some later stage as well – not a very healthy outlook! We place too much emphasis on statistics and, once again, in this way we inherit other people's beliefs. There are some highly respected doctors who, with the best of intentions, actually warn their patients to expect other symptoms in the syndrome to occur, thus making them almost inevitable. The power of the placebo[32] is well documented, but even more powerful is the effect of the 'nocebo'[33]. I would like to explore the way in which META-Health unpacks complex health issues into clear, understandable separate symptoms, so that the triggers and thought processes can be decoded from the illness.

Most often a name is given to a group of unrelated symptoms because they commonly occur together. This common, joint occurrence is often the only factor that links them. This is the case in illnesses such as influenza, lupus, fibromyalgia and even post-traumatic stress disorder (PSTD).

Let's examine why the symptoms of fibromyalgia may occur together in so many people. As with every META-Health analysis, each symptom will be separately investigated and finally put back together to form a fuller and more rounded picture.

---

32 A **Placebo** is 'a simulated or otherwise medically ineffectual treatment for a disease or other medical condition intended to deceive the recipient.' (Wikipedia)
33 'In medicine, a **nocebo** (Latin for "I shall harm") is a harmless substance that creates harmful effects in a patient who takes it.' (Wikipedia)

Fibromyalgia is commonly categorised by symptoms that include:

- Widespread musculo-skeletal pain, spasm, tightness and tenderness
- Fatigue – tiredness that is not relieved by sleep, poor sleep
- Poor cognition – brain fog and poor memory, inability to focus or concentrate
- Irritable bowel – bloating, abdominal pain, nausea, constipation alternating with diarrhoea
- Headaches – tension or migraine
- Sensitivities and allergies – to smells, bright lights, temperature, noise, food and medications
- Numbness - in the face, hands, feet, arms or legs
- Irritable bladder – increased frequency or urgency of urination
- Emotional state - feeling anxious or depressed.

Chronic fatigue syndrome (CFS) or myalgic encephalomyelitis (ME) features many of the above issues, but also includes other symptoms:

- Painful lymph glands – in the groin and under the arms
- Sore throat and flu-like symptoms
- Palpitations, dizziness and sweating.

Different organisations and doctors emphasise different symptoms for different diagnoses, but, in every case, a long list of separate, diagnosable illnesses gets grouped together under one or another label. Each of these individual symptoms may be difficult to manage on its own. In combination, they can become very debilitating, especially if we become trapped in our symptoms and degenerate into a state of chronic disease.

To be classified as suffering from either of these diseases - fibromyalgia or CFS/ME - a significant number of the criteria must be met. With diagnosis comes the label. This can be a life-saver for some people, but for others it is a life sentence. There are countless websites, books, magazines and support groups for each of these illnesses and, whereas this brings hope to many, it also risks becoming a lifestyle that holds the person trapped in the field of the illness group to which they have been ascribed. It can hardly be repeated too often that the greatest danger of this 'group diagnosis' is the blurring of the edges of the symptoms. This carries the assumption that all the symptoms belong together simply because they commonly appear together. If the symptoms and signs are not read individually, the messages they are sending us from the body cannot be understood. We stop listening to the body and become a victim of our labelling.

Break it down, before you have a breakdown

A doctor's diagnosis is always important for META-Health. It is important to understand what is actually happening in the body tissues to create a symptom. For example, many illnesses, such as liver jaundice, not just those that originate in the dermis or the epidermis, show their symptoms through the skin.

High blood pressure could be caused by narrowing arteries. Alternatively, it might be caused by something quite different, such as kidney disease, in which water retention in the blood is not is properly regulated and causes a build-up of water in the blood, increasing the pressure from the presence of more fluid.

Once we know what the body is doing and which tissue has changed, we can work out what happened to trigger the response. Every tissue responds independently and for its own reason - and there is always a reason.

The issue with syndromes, or collections of symptoms, is not that they are grouped together, but that in grouping them we may cease to look for the reason behind each individual symptom. There is a tendency to accept without demur that once we have enough symptoms in any group or syndrome, we are destined to get the others too - but why? Why is fibromyalgia so common and why do these symptoms so commonly occur together? There is no explanation from conventional medicine of why so many people get the same sets of symptoms and fall into the same patterns of dis-ease.

119

Although the *The Merck Manual of Diagnosis and Therapy*[34] states that the cause of fibromyalgia is 'unknown', there is widespread belief that the illness is stress-related and even associated with trauma. Most doctors advise using stress-management and thought-awareness tools, such as Cognitive Behavioural Therapy (CBT).

Using the META-Health model, we can break down the grouped symptoms to define the separate trigger of each component. This helps us to build an overall picture, including relevant, traumatic life events and stressors. Let us examine some of the main symptoms of fibromyalgia, according to their tissue, brain layer, theme and conflict, the tissue reaction and symptoms across the two phases of dis-ease.

It is worth recalling that cellular changes in the body and during the whole dis-ease process are meant only to be a brief, passing adaptation. The adaptation is intended to help us in situations of increased stress, but when that stress has passed we should enter into the second phase of repair and return to balance. Often, however, our thoughts re-trigger the original stressor, causing us repeatedly to recycle through the first, then the second, phase. Once in this loop, it depends on the individual whether they spend more time in the stress or repair phase of the process.

Although what follows is an overview of the general symptoms of fibromyalgia, I want to emphasise that each of these is an individual symptom in its own right. If you suffer from any of these symptoms, you can still use an individual META analysis to make sense of your own symptoms.

- *Widespread musculo-skeletal pain, spasm, tightness and tenderness*

    Association - The musculoskeletal system: all muscles, tendons, ligaments and joints are derived from the mesoderm germ layer and are associated with the **cerebral medulla.**

---

34 *The Merck Manual of Diagnosis and Therapy - Nineteenth edition*, Robert S. Porter MD (Editor-in-chief), Merck Sharp & Dohme Corp., New Jersey, USA, 2011

Theme - 'I am not strong enough or good enough to do something', depending on the part of the body and its function. For example, arms to hold on or to push away; legs to run towards or to flee; back to stand tall, to stand upright and to be myself.

- *Painful lymph glands in the groin and under the arms*

Association - The lymph glands are also derived from mesoderm and are associated with the **cerebral medulla.**

Theme - Fits the same theme of the cerebral medulla, but with the conflict 'I am redundant or worthless' or 'I am useless'.

The deeper the symptoms lie to the core of the musculo-skeletal system, the deeper is the perception of not being good enough. For example, problems in the tendons and ligaments indicate only a minor devaluation; muscles a suggest a deeper concern; bones imply an issue at a deeper level still; while bone marrow and associated changes at this level are very core. A deep level of 'I am not good enough' would manifest as 'I don't deserve to be alive'. When working with someone with leukaemia, especially a child, for example, we would look for an experience early in childhood, at birth or even *in utero* when the baby may have formed the 'belief' that they were not wanted. This can be as simple as a mother not feeling she is able or capable or even ready to have the child, resulting in the deep subconscious theme in the pre-born that 'I should not be here'.

Symptoms in first phase - In all these cases, we see a cell decrease in the stress phase when we do not experience any pain. However, becoming stuck in the stress phase with any of these triggers can lead to serious complications, such as muscle wastage or osteoporosis, for example. Hypermobility is also a symptom of the joints, tendons and ligaments being stuck in a programme in this phase.

121

Symptoms in the second phase - In all of these cases, whether lymph glands, tendons, ligaments, joints, muscles or bone, we see the symptoms of pain and discomfort in the regeneration phase - the second phase when the person feels better about the issue. However, in the case of chronic disease, there is a subconscious belief or trigger that prevents the client from moving out of the programme. This may be re-triggered either by external stimuli or by internal thoughts.

- *Irritable bowel - bloating, abdominal pain, nausea, constipation alternating with diarrhoea*

Association - The main organs of the digestive system are formed from the endoderm germ layer and are associated with the earliest part of the brain, the **brainstem**.

Theme - Digestion and survival. In our modern world, we process information as we would process food. Information comes in 'chunks'. These chunks are sometimes too big for us to take or break down, or perhaps sometimes there is information we don't want, or want but can't have. Our body responds as if this information were food - after all, it is sustenance for growth.

If we feel there is information that we cannot digest, our body makes an adjustment to help us to process it. This is particularly the case with the small intestine and the bowel, which absorb nutrients and take food into the body. The bowel also eliminates waste. The conflict associated with the bowel is 'indigestible anger'. This is more like an inner anger or frustration and is not to be confused with aggression. By this I mean that we are angry with someone or something and cannot understand what someone is doing, why they are doing it or why the situation is happening. Therefore, we hold onto the information to try to break it down so that we can absorb it - to make sense of it so that we can digest it.

Symptoms in the first phase - In the stress phase, when we are angry and cannot process the information, we hold onto it. The

122

body responds by holding onto whatever is in the bowel, because it understands the message 'I am not ready to let this go yet'. There is an increase of cells in the bowel to better digest the information. While in the bowel, however, more water is absorbed back into the body and the stools become dry and compact.

Symptoms in the second phase - In the resolution phase, we see the bowel relax and we are able to let go of the 'information'. This is the phase where the client would experience diarrhoea, bloating and discomfort. This is not just because the waste can now pass, but because the digestion and removal of the extra bowel cells takes place, so there is swelling and an accumulation of water that must be excreted once the healing has completed. During this phase, the *Candida albicans* fungus would be present to assist in degrading the extra bowel tissue.

If you experience the effects of *Candida albicans*, you may need to work back to identify and reconcile events where you have experienced these feelings of 'indigestible anger'. Although you may consider that the issue is resolved for most of the time, the presence of symptoms shows that the theme is still active and therefore you are still being triggered. This increases the activity in the repair, engaging more *Candida albicans* fungi.

- *Sore throat*

Association - The throat is part of the digestive system, where the food or 'chunk' enters. The pharynx is derived from the endoderm germ layer and is associated with the **brainstem**.

Theme - Digestion and survival. A change in the pharynx is triggered by a conflict of not being able to swallow something, to accept it or 'get it'. This could also be something that was promised and taken away again, such as a promotion.

123

Symptoms in the first phase - In the first phase, we see an increase of cells in the pharynx in order to grasp the 'chunk'. Initially this is not very noticeable, but tonsils may become enlarged if the first phase endures for some time.

Symptoms in the second phase - In the second phase, we see a decrease of cells with the help of a fungus or mycobacterium. This is most often when we have the symptoms of a sore throat with the apparent 'infection'.

- *Sensitivities and allergies - to smells, bright lights, temperature, noise, food and medications*

   Association - As with all META-Health analysis, it is necessary to know which tissue is involved so that we can understand the reaction. When we develop allergies or intolerances to foods or substances, it is because we have made an association with a particular substance during a trauma event. The very powerful subconscious mind takes a snapshot of everything in the outer and inner world at the point of trauma. It makes a record of everything, including the chemicals in the atmosphere, the smells that reach us, the sights we see, the foods in our systems and even the chemicals in our bloodstreams. It records everything and is ready to act again, should any of these aspects pose a threat in the future.

   The symptoms and the reaction of the body are particular to the trauma we experienced. A digestive disorder is related to processing information - as with coeliac disease, for example. A skin disorder would be related to contact, if it involved the epidermis, as in the case of dermatitis, or protection and integrity if it involved the dermis, as in the case of hives. Hay fever-type symptoms, such as rhinitis, are related to social annoyance and irritation.

   Once the association is made, the allergen will trigger the same response in future as it did in the first instance. Different people are affected in different ways by the same allergen - some get a runny nose, some itchy eyes, some a rash, some have breathing difficulties. This is because whatever the allergic reaction, it is based on what personal perceptions we experienced at the time of the original trauma. It may also be the case that if I *saw* something frightening it would affect my eyes, whereas if I *heard* something frightening it would affect my ears, and so on.

The most common allergic reaction for people with fibromyalgia is allergic rhinitis and sinusitis. The mucous membranes of the nose and sinuses are formed from ectoderm tissue and is associated with the **cerebral cortex**.

Theme - Territorial, social and contact. The conflict is social annoyance (something is strongly getting on my nerves) or the suspicion of danger (imagine a dog sniffing the air to find out what is going on).

Symptoms in the first phase - In the stress phase, the nasal and the sinus mucous membranes both thin in order to dilate the airways. This is to let more fresh air in, or obtain a larger sample of air to identify a smell. At this stage, we do not see many symptoms, since the breathing is better.

Symptoms in the second phase - In the regeneration phase, we see a repair of the mucous membranes, with swelling of the lining and viral activity in the repair of the tissue. This gives rise to the blocked and 'runny nose' symptoms. Sneezing dispels the pressure from a build-up of fluid and expels the allergen itself. Once the association has been made by the subconscious mind between the allergen and the trauma, the reaction is to expel it from the body whenever it is encountered. The symptom no longer needs to be triggered by an annoyance or the suspicion of a threat - the allergen is now the trigger representing the original trauma.

- *Irritable bladder - increased frequency or urgency*

  Association - The inner mucous membrane (mucosa) of the bladder is formed from the ectoderm germ layer and is associated with the 'new' brain, the **cerebral cortex**.

  Theme - Social, territorial, contact. The bladder mucosa is triggered by a conflict caused by an inability to recognise boundaries or limits, or to set boundaries.

  Symptoms in the first phase - In the stress phase, we see a cell decrease with a thinning of the bladder mucosa. The purpose is to make the bladder bigger to hold more urine, in order to mark one's territory. This ulceration can be painful and there is often an urgent impulse to urinate.

  Symptoms in the second phase - In the regeneration phase, there is an increase of cells and a repair of the bladder mucosa, with swelling and discomfort in the bladder and urethra and a strong urgency to urinate in the healing peak. To see a diagrammatic representation of the healing peak, go to *Natures two phases of disease*, chapter 4.

- *Numbness in the face, hands, feet, arms, legs or increased sensitivity to pain*

  Association - There seems to be no medical understanding of the numbness often associated with fibromyalgia. There are several theories, one being that there could be a link to MS. Multiple sclerosis affects the fatty tissue, the myelin sheath, that coats the axons of the nerves. The axons are nerve-cell extensions that transmit the signal. Fatty tissue is conductive, so it increases the speed of the nerve impulse. This tissue is formed from ectoderm tissue and is thus associated with the **cerebral cortex**.

Theme - Social, territorial, contact. There are different types of nerves - some for movement, some for sensitivity. A conflict in this case is to do with pain or unwanted contact.

Symptoms in the first phase - In the first phase, we see a cell decrease as the myelin sheath thins and fails to conduct the nerve impulse, causing desensitisation against the unwanted pain or contact.

Symptoms in the second phase - In the regeneration phase, we see a cell increase as the myelin sheath builds up again. In this phase also, we see a high level of sensitivity while repair is going on in the fatty tissue.

- *Headaches - tension or migraine*

There are different reasons, conflicts and physiological processes associated with a headache. Three of the main ones are:

- A fear of attack to the head, affecting the protective membrane (meninges) around the brain.
- A tension headache is often an intellectual self-devaluation: 'I am not good or clever enough' (a musculoskeletal conflict related to the cerebral medulla).
- Also, when an organ goes into repair and regeneration in the second phase, the corresponding relay also repairs. Water goes to the site in the brain to assist with this and the resulting oedema causes pressure in the brain, invoking a headache in the surrounding area. With a localised headache, it is possible to identify the position of the corresponding relay to the organ in regeneration.

- *Poor cognition - brain fog and poor memory, inability to focus or concentrate*

- *Fatigue – tiredness, flu-like symptoms*

  Poor cognition, tiredness and flu are common symptoms of the regeneration phase when we have come out of the 'fight or flight' mode and entered into rest and repair. The flu-like symptoms are caused by the body creating an optimal environment for bacteria and viruses to do their work.

- *Emotional states – feeling anxious or depressed*

> *Anxiety and depression associated with fibromyalgia is not simply related to coping with pain and illness. Like all other dis-ease, it is associated with specific triggers, or to be more accurate, a combination of specific triggers being active and running at the same time.*

Anxiety and depression associated with fibromyalgia is not simply related to coping with pain and illness. Like all other dis-ease, it is associated with specific triggers, or to be more accurate, a combination of specific triggers being active and running *at the same time*. They are always in specific areas of the brain and therefore create a particular pattern when viewed on a CT scan. These patterns look like a constellation, like stars in the sky. Both anxiety and depression are constellations.

I do not underestimate the difficulties of coping with severe or widespread pain, but this is not cause for the onset of anxiety or depression. Depression and anxiety are separate symptoms, just like the rest of the symptoms we have examined. And, just like the symptoms we have listed for fibromyalgia, we can trace the symptoms back to the root-cause event.

Association - When we have a specific change in behaviour, it is because two or more programmes have been triggered at the same time and in the case of anxiety or depression they are in the cerebral cortex.

128

We will cover this in more depth in the next chapter. However I will give you an outline here so as to complete the picture of the symptoms that are grouped under fibromyalgia.

Theme - Social, territorial, contact.

Anxiety - Powerlessness or helplessness, combined with fear of frontal attack, both being active at the same time.

Depression - A combination of inner-territory (such as being unable to define one's position) and outer-territory conflicts, with much greater emphasis (heavier traumatic experience) on outer-territory conflicts, such as territory fear, territory loss, territory anger, anger with family or territory marking.

Symptoms in the first phase - If both conflicts are active, a new behaviour (anxious or depressed) occurs.

Symptoms in the second phase - If one of the conflicts is resolved, the behaviour ceases.

The META-Health conclusion

Let us review the META meanings of each of these symptoms of fibromyalgia, together with the phases in which the symptoms appear. This builds a clear picture of how the symptoms appear and why.

- *Widespread musculo-skeletal pain, spasm, tightness and tenderness, and painful lymph glands in the groin and under the arms*

  Conflict or belief - 'I am not good enough or strong enough to do something'; 'I am redundant, worthless, useless.'

  Symptoms in stress - Weakening of the muscles, joints, tendons, ligaments.

Symptoms after stress - Aching muscles and joints, swelling and pain, stiffness and immobility, cramp and spasms in the healing peak.

- *Irritable bowel - bloating, abdominal pain, nausea, constipation alternating with diarrhoea*

  Conflict or belief - Indigestible anger and frustration - angry with someone or something and cannot understand what someone is doing, why they are doing it or why the situation is happening.

  Symptoms in stress - Constipation, bloating.

  Symptoms after stress - Diarrhoea.

- *Sore throat*

  Conflict or belief - Cannot swallow something, accept it or 'get it'. Something was promised and taken away again.

  Symptoms in stress - Thickness in throat.

  Symptoms after stress - Sore throat and infection.

- *Sensitivities and allergies - to smells, bright lights, temperature, noise, food and medications*

  Conflict or belief - 'Something is dangerous to me.' With rhinitis: 'this is annoying or irritating to me' or 'I must be prepared to sense danger.'

  Symptoms in stress - Clearer passageways for allowing air into the nasal passages.

  Symptoms after stress - Blocked nose, runny nose, bunged-up nose, sneezing.

- *Irritable bladder - increased frequency or urgency to urinate*

  Conflict or belief - Cannot recognise boundaries or limits, or unable to set boundaries.

  Symptoms in stress - Discomfort or pain in the bladder, with a strong urgency to urinate.

  Symptoms after stress - Swelling and discomfort in the bladder and urethra and a strong urgency to urinate at the healing peak.

- *Numbness in the face, hands, feet, arms, legs or increased sensitivity to pain*

  Conflict or belief - 'I do not want to feel pain or contact.'

  Symptoms in the first phase - A loss of sensitivity to pain and touch.

  Symptoms in the second phase - Increased sensitivity to pain and touch.

- *Headaches - tension or migraine*

  Conflict or belief - Tension headache: 'I am not good enough or clever enough.'

  Symptoms in stress - None.

  Symptoms after stress - Tension headache, tight scalp, aching and sensitive head and/or neck.

  Other symptoms after stress - Pressure headache, poor cognition, fatigue, flu-like symptoms.

- *Emotional - feeling anxious or depressed*

  Anxiety, conflict or belief - 'I am helpless, powerless', 'I am defenceless', 'I will be attacked, confronted', 'I cannot escape.'

  Symptoms in stress - Anxiety.

  Symptoms after stress - No anxiety, associated organs repair.

  Depression conflict or belief - 'I cannot define my inner world, protect myself, or define my position.' 'I have no control over my space.' 'I am afraid someone will attack me.' 'I will lose someone or something.' 'I am angry.' 'I cannot define my space.'

  Symptoms in the first phase - Depression.

  Symptoms in the second phase - No depression, associated organs repair.

The problem with stress management

From the META perspective, it is possible to see that most of these symptoms are in the second phase, that is, during regeneration. For the fibromyalgia sufferer, this means that symptoms will mostly appear when they are out of danger – when they come out of the 'fight or flight' phase and enter into rest and repair. This is a very new perspective for most people.

If we use a relaxation technique, such as breathing, meditation or EFT, to bring us out of stress, we enter into a state of rest and repair. Unless we fully understand what the body is doing, however, it is very possible that the symptoms we then experience will re-trigger us back into stress. For example, the belief that 'I am not strong enough or good enough' may be reinforced in the regeneration phase by musculo-skeletal weakness, aches and pain, together with tiredness and headache. This is a classic case of a chronic illness, in which we cannot exit the programmes running but remain stuck in the process. The symptoms themselves re-trigger us back into the process by reminding us of our underlying beliefs or fears.

This helplessness and lack of control will re-trigger the emotional aspects of anxiety or depression and it becomes increasingly difficult to take control of the situation or to tackle the individual symptoms.

Of course, it's important to manage our stress and to learn valuable techniques to bring us out of the 'fight or flight' response and our feelings of being overwhelmed. It is also important to learn new strategies to manage day-to-day stressors and ultimately to learn new perspectives. But, in my opinion, without visiting the original trauma to release the energy and to process the trapped emotion, stress management is still no more than symptom management. We can create new habits over time. We can make small steps towards greater changes and, eventually, it enters at a subconscious level, but it does take a long time and does not always alleviate the trigger.

META-Health enables us to go one step further: to make the specific connections and locate the triggering events, thoughts and beliefs that continue to re-trigger the body into a chronic dis-ease.

By examining the bio-logical reason for the META response (M – Meaningful, E – Emotional, T – Tissue, A – Adaptation), we can build a clear picture of a client's illness by including the missing link – the clear messages from the body-mind connection.

Is it at all possible that these separate symptoms of fibromyalgia occur together because common belief systems hold them together?

Events and traumas

In my experience, someone who has the symptoms of fibromyalgia has experienced a certain type of trauma and, most importantly, has formed specific beliefs and perceptions as a result. These events are still unprocessed, the beliefs are still active and the perceptions are still seen as real and true. These perceptions send messages to the body to adapt, in order to survive, and it is this process of adaptation that may result in dis-ease.

133

A META-Health coach works with a client and her/his symptoms to build a map that the client can navigate. Together client and coach decode the messages, identify the patterns and locate the traumas.

Beliefs and triggers

Although the traumatic experiences may be very individual, the theme of the beliefs is what makes the symptoms consistent in different people. Based on the META-Health analysis, I invite you to consider each of the following beliefs – frequently found among fibromyalgia sufferers.

> *Knowing that your body is looking after you, adapting to defend, protect and react for you, is a very different concept to the one that your body is a broken machine. This re-frame is usually the beginning of great changes for my clients in outlook, in lifestyle and in health."*

I would encourage anyone with fibromyalgia to test these core beliefs as a starting point to locate underlying patterns. I also challenge groups or organisations wishing to work with META-Health to gather some research in this area.

Out of 100 per cent, rate how true each of the following statements is for you (with 0 per cent being 'this is not at all true for me' and 100 per cent being 'this is completely true for me'). Be honest and answer quickly by tuning into your gut feeling, instead of trying to work out the answer consciously.

- I am not good enough
- I am not clever enough
- I am worthless
- I am useless
- I must be perfect
- People don't respect me
- I don't understand
- I can't let things go
- I am not in control
- I can't have what I want
- I can't accept things
- The world is a dangerous place
- I must sense danger
- Bad things will happen to me
- It's bad to say 'No' to people
- People take advantage of me
- I don't want to be hurt
- I will always get hurt

This list is by no means exhaustive and it goes only some way to identifying the main themes. Due to the nature of thought and perception, each person will have a very individual perspective on the way in which they make sense of the world. This type of analysis, however, does allow us to work holistically with the medical profession and the client in getting to the root cause of the issue. It is important to empower the individual, so that a full recovery and return to health is possible.

Knowing that your body is looking after you, adapting to defend, protect and react for you, is a very different concept to the one that your body is a broken machine. This re-frame is usually the beginning of great changes for my clients in outlook, in lifestyle and in health.

My own chronic fatigue

In the case of fibromyalgia, the most common META analysis finding is that it is the result of being stuck in a chronic healing cycle. This implies that the client has become stuck in the healing phase of multiple symptoms which constantly re-trigger the dis-ease. However, there are other illnesses that can cause fatigue, such as an underactive thyroid or underactive adrenal cortex. These have very specific triggers and reasons for a tissue response.

An overactive thyroid is triggered by a significant emotional event where someone believed 'I am not fast enough'. This could be fast enough to do something, get something or assimilate information. However, if the person believes 'I will *never* be fast enough', the thyroid will become underactive.

The adrenal cortex produces the stress hormone cortisol. We need small amounts of it to function properly. For example, I need a small boost of cortisol to get up in the morning. However, if I experience a trauma of 'moving in the wrong direction' or 'being thrown off course' my adrenal cortex will produce less cortisol to prevent me from heading off in the wrong direction. Imagine heading down the motorway and suddenly being unsure of where you are going!

My fatigue was caused by an event during my teaching career when I realised that I was in the wrong job. I was a good teacher, but the politics were just too much for me. One morning I experienced a traumatic event when my head of department believed accusations that I had spoken derogatorily about him behind his back in the presence of some sixth-form students. I was devastated that he could think I would do this and, at the same time as I experienced this, I remember feeling a deep sense of disappointment in my job and position. The voice in my head said, 'This is not for me'. I did not know it at the time, but this was the beginning of years of chronic fatigue.
META-Health helped me to make sense of this part of my life and to transform my health. Not only did it analyse the problem, but I found the direction in life that I *should* be pursuing and finally was able to shift into the second phase - the healing of this conflict.

7. Changing your mind

"You know how most illnesses have symptoms you can recognize? Like fever, upset stomach, chills, whatever. Well, with manic depression, it's sexual promiscuity, excessive spending, and substance abuse – and that just sounds like a fantastic weekend in Vegas to me!" **Carrie Fisher**[35]

It has been amazing to me that I can understand what my body is doing to help me. Understanding the root cause of my illness, relating the trauma to the dis-ease and the thought to its trigger has enabled me to bring about revolutionary changes in my life.

However, the greatest transformation I have experienced is coming to understand the phenomena that I was experiencing as mental and emotional imbalance or 'dis-ease'.

Was there a time when you were a little manic, a little hyperactive, and that very fact enabled you to complete a task that needed focused application? Or perhaps you were a little depressed, so you took yourself away for some quality 'me-time'? META-Health understands that all these natural responses serve a purpose: to maintain our energy and our health in a state of balance and to enable us to function in the face of constantly changing circumstances. Most of the time, these minor adaptations are so brief that we barely notice them as we go about our daily business.

If we adopt a structured understanding of how the body reacts, we are able to make logical connections between a tissue response and its triggers, such as in the example of the dilation of the bronchial tract to allow more

---

35 *Wishful Drinking*, Carrie Fisher, Simon & Schuster, New York, 2008

air into the lungs when confronted by a territorial fear. We can appreciate the highly intelligent way that these responses take place. Your body is not making mistakes. There is an instant change in your behaviour, a response in the organ tissue and a visible response in the brain - visible on a CT scan. In META-Health we refer to this simultaneous response as the 'organ-brain-psyche connection'. There is an instantaneous and simultaneous change in all these three areas, in order to cope with extra stress on the system.

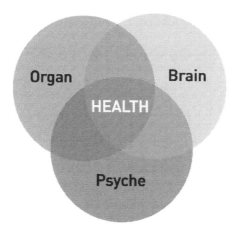

Fig.12 The biological, psychological, social connection

But what if this adaptation is not enough, what if there is an overload of information - just too many triggers operating at the same time?

Amazingly, the organ-brain-psyche connection has further adaptations that it can make in order to give us the best possible chance of survival. However, just like the specific organ programmes themselves, these psychological adaptations are only meant to be short-term changes to cope with an emergency situation. It is only when you become stuck in the process of adaptation that a problem is created.

If you don't change your mind ...

Because of our incredible capacity to adapt to situations, it would appear that if we are unable to change our minds and our thinking in the face of trauma or adverse stress, we enter into a new bio-logical programme that changes our minds for us.

These are also supposed to be short-lived adaptations, designed to assist us in resolving the issue. Just as becoming stuck in the two phases of a programme of tissue change becomes (a physical) dis-ease, so too a psychological change becomes (a mental) dis-ease if we cannot move through it and onwards to wellbeing. As with the symptoms of a physical disease, the amount of stress applied to the psyche is reflected in the severity and duration of the psychological reaction. A very severe acute incident or multiple, repeated incidents create a stronger psychological response.

The themes of psychological change
The four brain layers and their themes undergo specific behavioural and perceptual changes under stress. These changes are designed to maximise our potential to evade danger and to resolve issues as soon as possible. This response protects us on a number of levels - mostly by changing our perceptions and behaviours.

When we experience a traumatic event or a stimulus that reminds us of a traumatic event, we are triggered into a specific bio-logical programme designed to assist us in coping with the threat. Each type of conflict stimulates or 'hits' a different part of the brain and some conflicts stimulate many parts of the brain at the same time. The parts of the brain that are stimulated correspond directly to the organs that are required to increase their functions in order to react more effectively to the perceived threat. Because the brain is receiving specific information about the conflict in an ordered way, that information is received by different brain layers and on different sides (hemispheres) of the brain. We call these places in the brain 'impact points'. We have already examined the four brain layers:

- Brainstem (old brain)
- Cerebellum (old brain)
- Cerebral medulla (new brain)
- Cerebral cortex (new brain).

We know that for each brain layer there is an evolutionary theme, which defines the bio-logical adaptation that will be made by any associated organ tissue. To remind you, these are:

- Brainstem: 'digestion and survival of the species'
- Cerebellum: 'protection and integrity'
- Cerebral medulla: 'not strong enough or good enough'
- Cerebral cortex: 'social, territorial and contact'.

> *We know that for each brain layer there is an evolutionary theme, which defines the bio-logical adaptation that will be made by any associated organ tissue.*"

When multiple triggers impact on *both* the left and right brain hemispheres, there will be a change in behaviour that results in patterns - such as disorientation, emotional detachment, megalomania, depression, anxiety, aggression - according to the type of impact. Even so, each of these reactions is designed to protect us in some way.

It is reasonable to ask 'How can these psychological states be considered desirable or useful?' and 'How can they possibly constitute protection?'

Let's look at an example of impacts at each brain layer and examine the theme, to see how behaviour changes resulting from a multiple impact in left and right hemispheres would assist in resolving a specific situation.

Brainstem

Brainstem: associated with Endoderm Tissues
Theme: Digestion and Survival of the Species
Behaviour: Disorientation, Confusion, Short Term Memory Loss

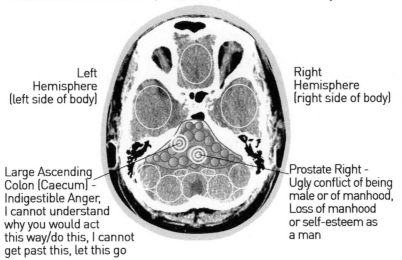

Left
Hemisphere
(left side of body)

Right
Hemisphere
(right side of body)

Large Ascending
Colon (Caecum) -
Indigestible Anger,
I cannot understand
why you would act
this way/do this, I cannot
get past this, let this go

Prostate Right -
Ugly conflict of being
male or of manhood,
Loss of manhood
or self-esteem as
a man

Fig.14 Two possible positions of triggers active in the brainstem creating disorientation

Theme *Digestion and survival of the species*
Conflicts arising in the brainstem are triggered by traumas associated with the most basic and primitive aspects of survival - food, breathing and reproduction. We also process information as if it were food, so our digestive system may be triggered to accommodate information in the same way as it does to these more basic drivers. We use expressions all the time that demonstrate our innate understanding of this metaphorical linkage: 'They rammed their opinion down my throat'; 'I'm not swallowing that'; 'I'm fed up to my back teeth'; 'I can't stomach it'; 'I couldn't let it go,' and so on.

Associated psychological changes *Disorientation and bewilderment, with space, time and oneself*

Imagine a sheep separated from its flock. She is alone and must survive, possibly without food or water, until her flock finds her again. Next to oxygen, the next most important thing for survival is water. She must have water for

141

survival. The body steps in to help the isolated sheep survive. Her kidney's collecting tubules automatically start to increase their cells in order to raise their effectiveness in retaining water.

In exactly the same way, a human trauma resulting in feelings of abandonment will trigger the kidney's collecting tubules to retain water as a defence against the perceived isolation. In other words, water retention occurs as a direct biological response to an emotional state of isolation and abandonment. Typical emotional expressions accompanying this state would be: 'I must do everything myself'; 'I am all alone in the world'; 'Everyone has deserted me'; 'No one cares for me'; 'I have lost everything.' The physical expression of this emotional state can be observed in the swollen ankles of the elderly, left in nursing homes.

Now imagine our lost sheep once again, wandering around looking for her flock, unable to find them and wandering further and further in her search. This is potentially more dangerous to her survival than staying where she is and waiting for the flock to find her. Now the sheep is confused; she can't remember or work out how to find the flock, so stops wandering and just stays put. This is the safest thing for the sheep to do, so that the flock has a better chance of catching up with her and she can avoid wandering into potential further danger.

In human terms, prolonged feelings of isolation and abandonment are likely to trigger both the left and right kidneys to respond. If the process continues and is not relieved, this will lead to a new, protective behaviour of disorientation and confusion, just as in the case of the lost sheep. Aged people living alone, with limited interpersonal contact, are much more likely to exhibit symptoms of disorientation and confusion than those who live in an environment where they are better integrated with family or friends, for example. And from a bio-logical point of view, it protects them from wandering or leaving the safety of the flock and heading into danger.

This protective behavioural change is also evident in the case of other combinations of conflicts across both the left and right hemispheres of the brainstem.

Case study *Colin's confusion and memory loss*

142

Colin was retired from his job as the successful head of department in a large, inner-city school. Now approaching his seventieth year, he was worried about his increasing tendency to forget things. Sometimes it extended to forgetting where he was and what he was supposed to be doing. Colin feared that he was experiencing the onset of Alzheimer's disease.

An investigation of Colin's past history revealed that his retirement had been accompanied by a great deal of trauma.

Colin's department had been recognised for its high standards and he was proud of this fact. Colin was livid, therefore, when a new teacher was hired for his department without his being consulted. He did not like the new man, who was surly and not personable. He could not understand why senior management had done this to his well-established and smooth-running team. He had felt so angry and betrayed by his senior management team that he took early retirement from a job to which he had devoted over 20 years. *Left hemisphere impact* Large intestine (colon).

Theme 'Indigestible anger or an ugly situation,' for example, a person is angry, does not understand or accept a situation, cannot process it or let it go.

Colin struggled to let go of his anger and still could not come to terms with the betrayal. Some years later, he was diagnosed with bowel cancer. Holding onto this deep anger, Colin's body had been acutely stimulated to assist in digesting the unacceptable situation.

Colin's anger with his situation at work was causing a lot of tension and upset with his younger wife at home. Colin was also exhibiting aggression to the point that his wife decided that she wanted him to leave. This was an enormous blow to Colin, since he was older than his wife and felt that he had been rejected because of his age.

Right hemisphere impact Prostate, right side.

Theme 'Loss of manhood.' This triggered a response in the right side of his prostate. The bio-logical purpose - to overcome the perceived loss of manhood by increasing cells to produce more ejaculate and 'spread his seed' - had remained unresolved. The result was emergence of an enlarged prostate.

Behavioural change It was during the time that these two programmes were active that Colin's episodes of short-term memory loss, confusion and disorientation began. In a simplistic, animalistic way, the purpose of the loss of memory would be to prevent Colin from dwelling on either of these issues, effectively helping him to forget about his emotional problems so that he could avoid re-triggering the conflicts and so prevent further bio-logical damage.

Cerebellum

Cerebellum: associated with Old Mesoderm Tissues
Theme: Protection and Integrity
Behaviour: Emotional Detachment

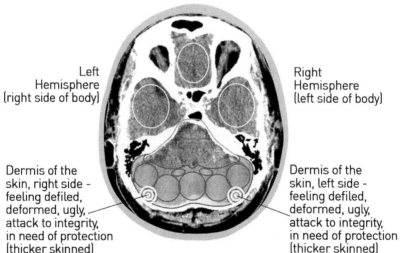

Left
Hemisphere
(right side of body)

Right
Hemisphere
(left side of body)

Dermis of the
skin, right side –
feeling defiled,
deformed, ugly,
attack to integrity,
in need of protection
(thicker skinned)

Dermis of the
skin, left side –
feeling defiled,
deformed, ugly,
attack to integrity,
in need of protection
(thicker skinned)

Fig.15 Two possible positions of triggers active in the cerebellum creating emotional detachment

Theme *protection and integrity*

Conflicts arising in the part of the brain called the cerebellum are triggered by trauma associated with the fear of attack to the person, or to the integrity.

Associated psychological changes *Emotional detachment, emotional burn-out, feeling 'dead inside' or 'emotionally cold'*

Case study *Sarah's acne and emotional detachment*
Sarah was a stereotypical 'stroppy teenager'. She appeared to have no interest in anyone or anything else. Her typical expressions were: 'I'm not bothered'; 'I don't care what you think'; 'I couldn't give a damn.' Investigation of Sarah's background demonstrated the link to her underlying issues.

As Sarah approached puberty, she began to care what her friends thought of her and, even more importantly, what the opposite sex thought of her. Her parents started to remind her that she was 'a young lady now' and should act like one. Sarah became worried about her looks and a very embarrassing incident that occurred in front of her school friends made things worse for her. This incident triggered the onset of her acne, when the dermis tissue of her skin thickened in order to 'protect' her from what people might think about her. She felt that she needed to be 'thicker-skinned' to cope with that fear. Sarah developed acne under the skin, in red, painful lumps.

In the META-Health analysis in Chapter 5, you will recall that we tested Amy's laterality (which hand and side was more dominant) in order to establish how she interpreted the world. The dominant side would relate to equal partners, friends and carer and her non-dominant side would relate to her nurturing relationships.

Left and right hemisphere impact Sarah developed acne on both sides of her face because she was triggered both by what her parents said to her and by what her friends might think of her. She cares what everybody thinks of her. This means that both the left and the right hemispheres of the cerebellum have active conflicts running at the same time.

Behavioural change Because both sides of her brain are running active conflicts, Sarah assumes a new kind of behaviour. This behaviour is designed to protect her from the anxiety aroused by her situation. Now she enters a phase when she no longer cares what anyone thinks. So, for those of you who are used to dealing with difficult teenagers, think about the deeper,

145

underlying insecurity that drives this behaviour. It is a psychological protective mechanism designed to assist a highly sensitive person to be less sensitive, so that they can continue to function despite their active stress triggers. This is also the case for other conflicts arising in the cerebellum.

Cerebral medulla

Cerebral Medulla: associated with New Mesoderm Tissues
Theme: Movement and Strength
Behaviour: Megalomania

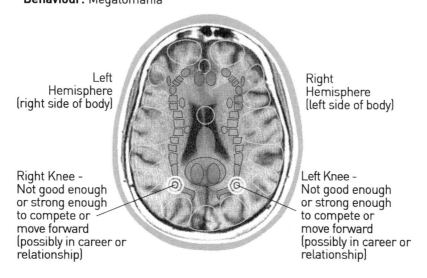

Left
Hemisphere
(right side of body)

Right
Hemisphere
(left side of body)

Right Knee –
Not good enough
or strong enough
to compete or
move forward
(possibly in career or
relationship)

Left Knee –
Not good enough
or strong enough
to compete or
move forward
(possibly in career or
relationship)

Fig.16 Two possible positions of triggers active in the cerebral medulla creating megalomania

Theme Strength and movement

This brain layer is associated with the musculo-skeletal system and with movement and strength. If someone has a traumatic experience in which they feel that there are not strong enough or good enough to do something, a programme in this brain layer and the associated part of the body will begin. The purpose is to ensure that the area of the body implicated by the trauma will emerge stronger at the end of the process to cope with any future challenges.

146

With this brain layer, left or right dominance is also relevant.

Just to recap at this point, we can test the way in which a person makes sense of the world and metaphorically interprets interactions with people and situations by determining which is their dominant and non-dominant side. This is because conflicts regarding a career, equal person or relationship will be expressed on the dominant side, while conflicts regards a nurturing relationship will express on the non-dominant side. (In Chapter 5 we already described a simple hand-clapping method for checking hemispherical dominance).

Associated psychological changes *Megalomania*

Case study *Robin's weak knees and megalomania*

Robin was the sort of person who always knew best. No one could tell him anything that he didn't know better himself. He appeared to possess an inflated sense of self-importance. He was convinced that he was (and had to be) the best, the fastest and the most intelligent. He found it impossible to work with others whom he considered beneath him in all these areas.

Robin had particularly weak knees. Both knees troubled him and had been causing him pain for some time.

In discussion, it emerged that at school Robin had felt that he could not compete with the other children in his class. A traumatic event during a sports tournament, when he had come in last and everyone, including the teachers, had laughed at him, triggered a belief that 'I am not good enough to compete with the others.' He felt that he would never be as good as his teachers or as good as the other children.

This belief began a programme in both his knees to make them stronger and more able to compete. The knees provide us with the ability to move forwards and to be flexible in changing direction and acting fast. When we are competing against others, the knees are vital to being able to react quickly to beat and outshine an opponent.

147

Behavioural change This programme, as we have said, is designed to assist in coping with low self-worth and low self-esteem. Rather than endure such low self-worth that you dare not go out into the world for fear that you are 'not good enough', it is far better for you, bio-logically speaking, to believe that you can achieve anything. That way, you get to go out and you have the drive to succeed. In fact, people who believe themselves to be the best have often set out to prove that they are, thus naturally resolving their issue with being good enough to compete.

Cerebral cortex

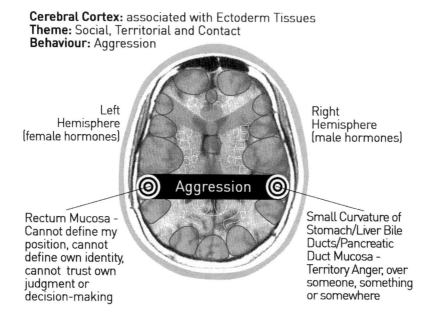

Cerebral Cortex: associated with Ectoderm Tissues
Theme: Social, Territorial and Contact
Behaviour: Aggression

Left Hemisphere
(female hormones)

Right Hemisphere
(male hormones)

Aggression

Rectum Mucosa - Cannot define my position, cannot define own identity, cannot trust own judgment or decision-making

Small Curvature of Stomach/Liver Bile Ducts/Pancreatic Duct Mucosa - Territory Anger, over someone, something or somewhere

Fig.17 Two specific positions of triggers active in the cerebral cortex creating aggression

Theme *Social, territorial, contact*

This is a highly developed and complicated part of the brain. Many different adaptive behaviours may be involved when the cerebral cortex is triggered in both the left and right hemispheres. Depending on the traumas that someone

148

has experienced and, therefore, which parts of the cortex are active, a very specific new behaviour may be triggered.

It is always worth remembering that the severity of a particular behaviour is proportional to the severity of the traumatic experience, or the energy that is built up in the system. This can be a single, very acute incident, or many repeated triggers or lesser incidents over time.

Associated psychological changes *There are very specific changes in behaviour associated with the cerebral cortex, such as anxiety, depression, bipolar disorder, anorexia, bulimia, self-harming or aggression.*

A few years ago I suffered from 'aggression'. I was drinking a lot to escape my life situation and this meant that I did not have very good control over my emotions. Aggression is not just an angry outburst; it is the uncontrollable need to lash out violently either verbally or physically. It is the instant and sudden flip from being rational and in control to being totally out of control. It is a rage that comes from nowhere.

There are two types of trauma that create this kind of aggressive reaction. Like all these behavioural examples, the two different traumas may happen together, or they may happen separately, but once they are there and both active at the same time, a new behaviour will be expressed. Once more, the biological intention is to protect the person from a repeat of the same trauma as initiated the response.

The earliest event I have traced back in my own case is the event that I have already mentioned in Chapter 5[36] regarding David and the colouring book when I was four years' old. Those traumas gave rise to the following conflicts:

Right hemisphere *Territory anger - anger over something that I considered to be mine as well as the perception that someone had taken or damaged my property.*

---

36 See Chapter 5, *David and the Colouring Book*

Left hemisphere Self-identity/decision-making, cannot define my position: thoughts such as 'I cannot express myself'; 'You are not taking me seriously'; 'You don't believe me'; 'You are not listening to or validating me'; 'I can't trust myself.'

There is an interesting duality about this conflict: when the outer-territory anger is predominant or has more energy, there is a more depressive aspect to the aggression. Because you cannot control your outer world, you turn more **inwards,** into yourself. This depressive aspect results in aggressive internal self-talk and, in strong or extreme cases, self-harming.

When the conflict of not being able to define your position or express your self-identity is greater than the outer-territorial anger, you must try to take some control over your *outer* world. The aggression is turned **outwards** and you will become more outwardly aggressive towards others. Where you were previously unable to explain yourself in order to affect events, you are now full of energy that wants to express itself in outward action. The greater the trauma of not being able to define your position, the more energy is stored in the system and needs to 'burst' out!

The only response left

The four-year-old me saw David writing in my best colouring book. He had defaced it. I told my mum, who said 'Aw, he's not doing any harm', and did nothing to stop him or reconcile the situation. I was angry and utterly helpless to make my position clear. At this I flipped and in desperation kicked David in the shin. This was an instinctive response; there was no time to decide whether this was a good or bad thing to do. During that moment of trauma, the 'UDIN (Unexpected, Dramatic, Isolating, No strategy) moment', both conflicts were activated together - one on the left side of the brain and one on the right.

The new behaviour that was intended to help me in this situation was to express the energy of the conflicts outwardly, in order to take control over my outer territory and to compensate for having less control over my inner territory (my emotional position).

Of course, I have not spent the rest of my life kicking people in the shins or having outbursts of rage. However, because these traumas had never been revisited and resolved, the possibility for triggering the same feeling was always there under the surface. So, even though the event had passed and was forgotten to my conscious mind, I had become hyper-vigilant to the prospect of people damaging my things and, more importantly, to people not validating my feelings. When, later in life, I found myself in situations where I felt I was not being understood, my frustration became a growing concern. At the first sign that my partner was not validating my position or feelings - even if I was consciously aware their actions were not intentional - this deep, subconscious trigger would flip inside. The resulting emotion was rage.

Through analysing my aggressive behaviour using the META-Health model, I was able to identify the conflicts that had created this pattern. This helped me to pinpoint the theme of the events I was looking for: territory anger and 'cannot define my position'. Using EFT and Matrix Reimprinting, I was able to go back by means of the more recent triggers in my current relationship to find the earliest traumatic memory that had the same theme and work on it. Using the same techniques, I was able to resolve the traumas and release the energy from those events. I would say that I have mostly resolved this issue by now. Nonetheless, if I feel someone is not validating my feelings or is misunderstanding my motives, I do feel a slight rising of energy inside. Because of the understanding and foresight that I have gained, that energy passes swiftly. If for any reason it does not, however, I have a choice of energy therapy tools to release it.

That said, the purpose is never to avoid our emotions, but to understand them and listen to them. This is a normal processing of emotions.

If I am sarcastic or snappy with my husband, I reflect on what I may have concluded from an exchange or a response and I am quickly able to see the connection between the current situation and my own habitual thought patterns. This gives me an immediate opportunity to process my emotions, to apologise, and to explain that I was triggered, that it's my own stuff and

151

that I will deal with it. It is such a different way of seeing the world. Being responsible for my own thoughts and reactions has transformed my life. I am now the person I want to be in the world.

Releasing judgment and finding the gift
There is great knowledge in these messages from the body.

> *Life experiences, even those encountered in your mother's womb before you are born, are recorded and stored in your subconscious mind. This information is held in your energy field as your reference for how to make sense of the world.*

Life experiences, even those encountered in your mother's womb before you are born, are recorded and stored in your subconscious mind. This information is held in your energy field as your reference for how to make sense of the world. Those experiences, most certainly until you are six years' old, create your ground rules for perceiving the world around you - to sense danger, to function in society and ultimately to develop and become an enlightened being. We each have our life lessons to learn. Embracing your emotions and the messages from your body will point the way to what you need to learn.

The events of our lives too can become signposts on the journey. When we experience pain or suffering, it is difficult to stand back from negative judgment because these are generally considered 'undesirable' states. After all, who really wants to be miserable?

But what if we were to look at these states from another perspective? What if it were the case that we always receive just what we need, in order to help us to *evolve*? There is a lesson in every experience; there is always an opportunity for growth. If we can decode the messages and understand the lessons, we can learn and grow.

We constantly seek balance. We seek peace and harmony in our bodies and our minds. The adaptations and adjustments to our systems help us to manage

152

stress, so that the energy surrounding traumatic events can be processed and our equilibriums can be restored. An excess of any kind is not balance - even an excess of happiness.

It is my belief that when we find peace, we are in harmony. If this is through change and adaptation, then we have grown. We have evolved. All of the physiological and psychological changes that we have mentioned so far are responses to stress. However, what was once initially a stressor may also be a great learning opportunity, once it has been understood and processed. It is only *unprocessed* stress that puts weight on the system and risks damaging the body.

As the saying goes, 'What doesn't kill us makes us stronger.'

In order to become stronger, you must go through the two phases, not get stuck in them. If you are stuck in a dis-ease process, it indicates that you did not resolve your traumatic event and have yet to benefit from the challenge of growing stronger as a result of it. META-Health not only shows you where you are in the struggle, it even shows you what you are struggling with.

The butterfly's struggle

A man found a cocoon of a butterfly. One day a small opening appeared in the cocoon. The man sat and watched the butterfly for several hours as it struggled to force its body through that little hole.

Then it seemed to stop making any progress. It appeared that it had gotten as far as it could and could go no further. So the man decided to help the butterfly. He took a pair of scissors and snipped off the remaining bit of the cocoon.

The butterfly then emerged easily. But it had a swollen body and small, shrivelled wings. The man continued to watch the butterfly because he expected that, at any moment, the wings would enlarge and expand to be able to support the body that would contract in time.

Neither happened! In fact, the butterfly spent the rest of its life crawling around with a swollen body and shrivelled wings. It never was able to fly.

What the man, in his kindness and haste, did not understand was that the restricting cocoon and the struggle required for the butterfly to get through the tiny opening were nature's way of forcing fluid from the body of the butterfly into its wings so that it would be ready for flight once it achieved its freedom from the cocoon.

Sometimes struggles are exactly what we need in our lives. If we were allowed to go through our lives without any obstacles, it would cripple us. We would not be as strong as we could have been. We could never fly!
Unknown author

If an organism has to make a change for survival, it will adapt to adverse conditions and will become stronger as a result. If those conditions persist, it will continue to adapt until the change becomes permanent. This is the process of evolution.

Not all struggle is detrimental. Not all change is bad and not all adaptation is dis-ease. Some change is evolution and a necessary development of the species towards balance and harmony in the face of changing circumstances. Sometimes a new equilibrium must be struck so that, as the old ways die, a new way can be established.

Further developments in the cerebral cortex
It cannot be denied that the psychological aspect of the META-Health model is a complex one. Now we are ready to look into a further area of study, related to the left and right hemispheres of the cerebral cortex. It concerns the balance of male and female hormones and is an area of great personal interest to me. Understanding this aspect may provide us with some very useful insights into commonly observed patterns of behavioural change.

To appreciate this model, we must remember that we are observing very fundamental, animalistic bio-logical responses in humans. We have a natural pre-disposition to function in male and female biological roles for the survival and protection of the species.

> *Not all struggle is detrimental. Not all change is bad and not all adaptation is dis-ease. Some change is evolution and a necessary development of the species towards balance and harmony in the face of changing circumstances. Sometimes a new equilibrium must be struck so that, as the old ways die, a new way can be established."*

The left hemisphere of the cerebral cortex controls the production of female hormones and the right hemisphere controls the production of male hormones. This is the case in both men and women. Men are biologically predisposed to react in a 'masculine' way, as the hunter and provider. This means that a man will normally interpret a territorial conflict as a masculine, 'outer territory' conflict where he must protect and defend his territory (including his land, his things, his partner and his family) from predators.

A woman's biological task is to have babies and to tend the nest. For this reason, she is predisposed to react in a 'feminine' way, with the emphasis on her 'inner territory' – her ability to understand what is going on, to communicate and to be the child bearer. We are talking purely from a biological position here and I make no judgment about gender roles or 'equal opportunities'. We are talking about early evolutionary conditions dating back to the dawn of humanity, when women remained in the nest to have and to nurture babies, while the men hunted for food and protected the nest.

Because of this background, men and women are hard-wired to perceive situations differently and therefore to adapt and respond to situations differently. There are five areas on the left (female) side and five areas on the right (male) side of the cerebral cortex; these areas affect the way in which the cortex controls hormones in the body. If one of the areas is triggered or stimulated by a territorial conflict (trauma), a message is sent to suppress the production of hormones controlled by that side of the brain. This will induce a slight change in the balance of hormones and in the person's perception of the situation.

We will stay with the example of a right-handed man and a right-handed woman to avoid confusion, since the sequence is slightly different for left-handed men and women.

When a right-handed man perceives a territorial threat, it will trigger a response in the right hemisphere of his cerebral cortex. As well as the organ-brain reaction, a message will be sent to suppress the production of male hormones. His next territorial perception and response will therefore be more feminine.

When a right-handed woman perceives a territorial threat, it will trigger a response in the left hemisphere of her cerebral cortex. This will cause a reaction in a specific organ, but also sends a message to suppress the production of female hormones. Her next territorial perception and response will therefore be more masculine.

The bio-logical purpose of both of these changes is demonstrated in the following story of the couple and the burglar.

The couple and the burglar

A husband and wife were fast asleep in bed one night when they were suddenly awoken by a loud noise downstairs. The man leaped out of bed, grabbed a nearby baseball bat and set off downstairs, in his pyjamas, to see what the commotion was. The wife hurried into the children's bedroom to huddle with them beside the bed, in case the danger came upstairs. The brave and perhaps foolish man came face to face with a fearsome burglar, who proceeded to beat the man up before making off with his TV and DVD player. On hearing the commotion downstairs, the woman was very afraid, but could not cry out for fear of attracting violence.

Both the man and the woman experienced their initial territorial traumas.
The man perceived a threat to his territory - his house, his family, his belongings - and so experienced a male, territory-fear conflict. He needed to square up to the invader, so this triggered the part of his cerebral cortex on the right hemisphere (the male side), associated with the bronchial mucous

membranes. This is because the mucous membranes in the bronchi thin in the event of a territory fear, in order to allow more air in and be ready for a fight. This thinning occurs in the stress phase.

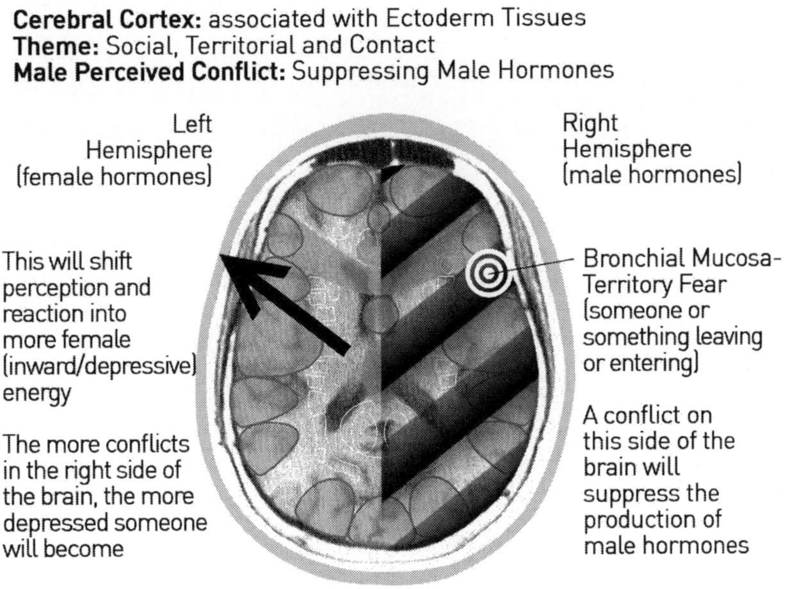

Cerebral Cortex: associated with Ectoderm Tissues
Theme: Social, Territorial and Contact
Male Perceived Conflict: Suppressing Male Hormones

Left Hemisphere (female hormones)

Right Hemisphere (male hormones)

This will shift perception and reaction into more female (inward/depressive) energy

Bronchial Mucosa- Territory Fear (someone or something leaving or entering)

The more conflicts in the right side of the brain, the more depressed someone will become

A conflict on this side of the brain will suppress the production of male hormones

Fig.18 Conflict of territory fear in the right hemisphere suppressing male hormones

Unfortunately, the man failed to resolve his territory-fear conflict because he was defeated. This left him with an active conflict in the right hemisphere. The right hemisphere (associated with the bronchial mucous membranes) is the side that also controls the production of male hormones. When the conflict remains active, the production of hormones is inhibited. This inhibition of hormones will subtly change his perception and behaviour.

The woman was unable to cry out to raise help to protect herself and her children - this is a female, territory-fear conflict. This conflict causes a thinning of the larynx's mucous membrane, in order to dilate the throat and allow for better breathing and the ability to scream. The area associated with the larynx's mucous membrane - also associated with not being able to cry out - is in the left hemisphere of the cerebral cortex. Because her

157

natural strategy of crying out for help and alerting others to danger could not be achieved, the woman is left with an unresolved conflict in her left hemisphere. Her left hemisphere is the side that controls the production of female hormones and this is now inhibited. Suppressing the release of female hormones will change her perception and her behaviour in the future.

Cerebral Cortex: associated with Ectoderm Tissues
Theme: Social, Territorial and Contact
Female Perceived Conflict: Suppressing Female Hormones

Left
Hemisphere
(female hormones)

Right
Hemisphere
(male hormones)

Larynx Mucosa -
Shocking fear,
fright,
speechless

This will shift
perception and
reaction into
more male
(outward/manic)
energy

A conflict on
this side of the
brain will
suppress the
production of
female hormones

The more conflicts
in the left side of
the brain, the more
manic someone
will become

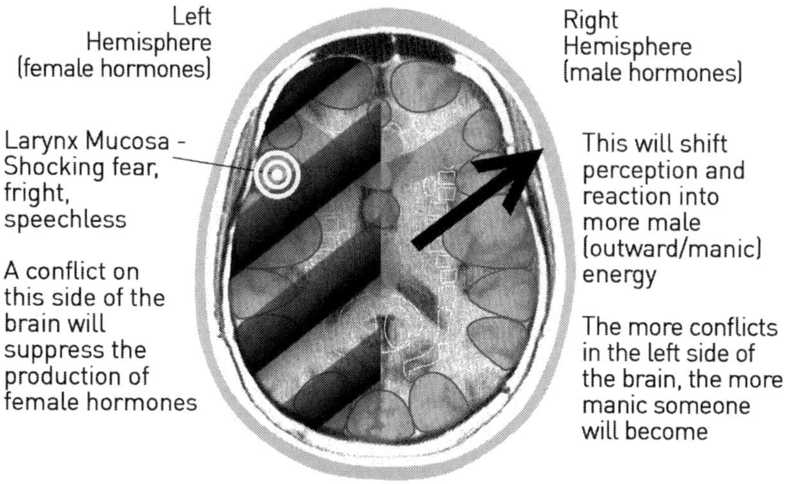

Fig.19 Conflict of fear / fright / speechless in the left hemisphere suppressing female hormones

A few weeks later, the couple received their insurance money and replaced their stolen goods with nice, new ones. They stacked the boxes outside by the bin, which allowed the observant burglar to see that they now have new equipment. Back in bed that night, the couple heard a noise downstairs ... What do you think happened?

The man (who is now reacting with a more feminine energy because of his reduction in production of his male hormones) slides down under the covers, thinking, 'Well, I'm not going down there again; I got beaten up last time; I will wait here until he has gone.' The woman on the other hand (who is now reacting with a more masculine energy because of her reduced production of female hormones) thinks, 'I'm not having this stranger coming into my home, threatening my family and taking our things.' She grabs the baseball bat and storms downstairs to chase away the burglar!

In both cases, the active, unresolved conflict created a new behaviour that assisted in resolving the issue next time in a different way.

Although this is a simple story, it demonstrates the way in which conflicts in the cerebral cortex can affect our perceptions and our behaviours. The more conflicts that impact on one side of the brain, the more hormone production on that side will be inhibited and the greater the shift in perception and behaviour.

> *In both cases, the active, unresolved conflict created a new behaviour that assisted in resolving the issue next time in a different way.*

I am in a unique position because I have experimented with my hormone balance to extremes. I was born a woman, but have undergone gender realignment and have injected testosterone for the last fifteen years. I have always done it with the intention to remain somewhere between the genders, rather than to go to the other extreme and become a man. The gift I now have from this experience is that I am better able to understand the connection between my perceptions and my behaviours. Using the META-Health model, it is even possible to locate early conflicts that may have caused the subtle shift in hormones, early on in my life, that led me to regard gender difference as an issue in the first place.

The evolution of gender

There is much research and evidence that goes some way in explaining how life experiences can alter our views of the world. However, I must make the argument here that there is no judgment attached to gender roles, gender identity or sexual preference. We have an enormous ability to adapt to our surroundings and to evolve. Changes of this kind give way to the rainbow spectrum of female, lesbian, gay, male and transgender differences. If we take the argument of nature versus nurture, I would say that it is now moot, since we have scientific evidence, through the study of epigenetics, that our environment affects the readout of our genes[37] and that we also inherit thoughts and beliefs from our families and primary carers. This means that we are an accumulation of both factors - events before our birth and events since.

If we entertain the concept that we, as a species, are constantly seeking balance and equilibrium, it seems natural to me that we adapt to survive and to function as part of the group, as well as to fulfil our personal potentials. To do this we must adapt to bring balance. We seek to achieve and to maintain personal and social harmony. There is plenty of evidence, for example, of birds and animals naturally establishing gay relationships[38]. This maintains balance in the group and in the population.

I believe that developments throughout the world regarding gender and sexuality are evolutionary. The evolution of gay, lesbian, bisexual, trans-sexual, and transgendered people is a necessary development in human relationships and in personal and social harmony. We both personally and societally (and even globally) have a constant shifting polarity of male/female energy and this is regulated by a shift in the energy of individuals en masse. I have experienced life in both gender roles and am now equipped with a deep understanding of both genders on a biological, personal and social level. I see my ability to be a 'gender chameleon' as the greatest gift. It affords me the deepest sense of rapport and connection with people and I am grateful for the events in my life that may have contributed to my taking this life path.
I do recognise, however, that people like me are ahead of the trend. There is still much confusion and fear around the emergence of pan-gender[39] and pan-sexuality[40],which many people still do not understand and so find hard to accept. All any of us can do is to work on our own issues, so that we may learn the lessons we are here to learn. Each trauma we release, each blockage

---

37 *The Biology of Belief - Unleashing the Power of Consciousness, Matter & Miracles*, Bruce H. Lipton PhD, op. cit.
38 See, for example, *Biological Exuberance - Animal Homosexuality and Natural Diversity*, Bruce Bagermihl PhD, St Martin's Press, New York, 1999
39 Pangender: *A person who does not conform to binary gender standards. Someone who identifies as neither male nor female, but instead a third gender.* (www.urbandictionary.com)
40 *Pansexuality, or omnisexuality, is sexual attraction, sexual desire, romantic love, or emotional attraction toward people of all gender identities and biological sexes.* (Wikipedia)

we free and each lesson we learn brings us closer to knowing that we are all connected and that what we do to each other we do to ourselves.

Wouldn't life be different if we could accept that each person is doing the best that they possibly can, with the resources they have available to them at any time?

Depression and being bipolar

The same hormonal mechanism in the cerebral cortex that creates a shift in gender perception can also create a shift in mood that results in depression or bipolar disorder.

This is another complex area, but, based on the research and as a general rule, people who are right-side dominant will experience multiple conflicts on the same side of the brain, causing them to become either increasingly manic or increasingly depressed, whereas those who are left-side dominant will experience conflicts on both left and right sides of the brain, depending on how much trauma is already stored on each side.

For a right-side-dominant person, the more traumatic events or re-triggers the person experiences, the more energy goes into the already most heavily affected side of the brain. If it is the right side of the brain (governs the production of male hormones), the person will inhibit production of male hormones more and more and turn more and more 'inwards'. Similarly, if it is the side of the brain that governs production of female hormones, those hormones will be inhibited and the person will become more and more manic and 'outwards'. This can happen to men or women.

For example, Andrea is a right-hand-dominant girl. She experienced a trauma when her mother told her off for doing something which Andrea had thought was a good idea. This caused a self-identity ('cannot define my position', 'cannot trust my decision') conflict, which we know to occur on the left side of the cerebral cortex. Andrea then experienced a territory-anger conflict when her mother painted her bedroom a colour that she hated, against her expressed wish. This second conflict was much greater than the first and

161

impacted on the right (male) side of the cerebral cortex. Because this second trauma was greater, there was a greater suppression of the male hormones. This made Andrea more feminine, more 'inwards' and more depressed. The bio-logical purpose was 'to retreat and regroup'. Although the strategy is designed to avoid similar conflicts, if Andrea were to experience a similar conflict, as a right-side-dominant person, she would become further 'inwards' and more depressed.

Left-side-dominant people adopt a different strategy. This is because the severity of the conflicts that they receive can switch to either side of the brain. The point of impact will depend on the amount of trauma already stored in each brain hemisphere. The change in hormones in the left and right sides balances like a see-saw and each new conflict could tip the energy one way or the other.

If the right hemisphere becomes more overwhelmed with trauma (such as territory fear, anger or loss), this will inhibit production of male hormones and send the person more inwards to retreat, exactly as would a right-side-dominant person with depression. However, a left-side-dominant person can also be triggered by conflicts in the left hemisphere (such as territory shock, territory fear, for example 'can't cry out' or 'cannot define my position') and, if the amount of energy becomes greater in the left side, the balance will flip and production of female hormones will be more inhibited. This will cause the person to become more manic and 'outwards'.

Eating disorders and self-harming

Using this information, we are able to make sense of the conflicts involved in anorexia, bulimia and manic or depressive types of aggression. All these different psychological and behavioural changes share a common conflict in the right hemisphere: 'territorial anger', most often affecting the small curvature of the stomach. This can cause an ulcer or discomfort and bloating in the stomach, which would in part explain the desire not to eat or retain food in the stomach. With bulimia, a 'fear/disgust' conflict triggers a drop in blood sugar, hence the craving for something sweet, followed by purging due to the ulcer. Anorexia can be caused by a number of different inner-territorial conflicts in the left hemisphere, combined with territory anger; however, in my experience, I have always found that there is a 'cannot define position' conflict, which explains the commonality between those with anorexia and self-harming.

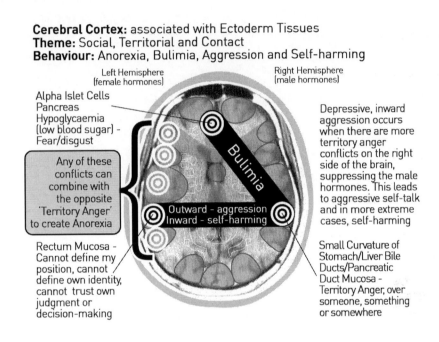

Cerebral Cortex: associated with Ectoderm Tissues
Theme: Social, Territorial and Contact
Behaviour: Anorexia, Bulimia, Aggression and Self-harming

Left Hemisphere
(female hormones)

Right Hemisphere
(male hormones)

Alpha Islet Cells
Pancreas
Hypoglycaemia
(low blood sugar) -
Fear/disgust

Any of these conflicts can combine with the opposite 'Territory Anger' to create Anorexia

Bulimia

Outward - aggression
Inward - self-harming

Depressive, inward aggression occurs when there are more territory anger conflicts on the right side of the brain, suppressing the male hormones. This leads to aggressive self-talk and in more extreme cases, self-harming

Rectum Mucosa -
Cannot define my position, cannot define own identity, cannot trust own judgment or decision-making

Small Curvature of Stomach/Liver Bile Ducts/Pancreatic Duct Mucosa -
Territory Anger, over someone, something or somewhere

Fig.20 Diagram of the cerebral cortex showing the connection between anorexia, bulimia, aggression and self-harming

I have used this model with great success to fathom the complex thoughts and processes of eating disorders, aggression, depression and bipolar disorder. If you have either of these illnesses, how does it make you feel to know that there is a clearly defined reason for the way in which your mood swings or your deep feelings of despair are triggered? Having this information allows a 'plan of action' for even the deepest and most complex of these issues. Working with your doctor, as well as with this META view of your symptoms, empowers you to take control of your patterns and behaviours. For me, it was a huge turning point in my life.

The energy of stress

If we look at balance in energetic terms, we must process energy and allow it to flow in order to return to equilibrium. As we have seen with the two phases of dis-ease, we only have a physical or psychological illness if there is a blockage that causes the information to be either malformed or unprocessed. The message gets stuck, as if the energy enters the system, but does not leave. This is what happens with the freeze response when the energy of the trauma is embodied.

> *Wouldn't life be different if we could accept that each person is doing the best that they possibly can, with the resources they have available to them at any time?*

When you learn to decode the messages from your body, the process becomes a fluid one - trauma is processed and becomes an opportunity to grow stronger, while emotions become your navigation system.

If someone is not exhibiting physical symptoms, but has an undesired behaviour pattern, we can still use this same information to work our way back to the root cause, by understanding how psychological dis-ease is constructed from specific conflicts. Psychological changes, just like physical changes, happen by degrees and are proportional to the amount of stress at the time of trauma or re-triggering. It is possible to release stress from the system and to understand the fundamental message, using newly learned information. I have been pleased to learn the deeper messages from my most painful experiences. I still have work to do, but at least now I can read the signs. I am not afraid to explore where the rabbit hole goes.

8. Are you trigger-happy?

"There is no fixed physical reality, no single perception of the world, just numerous ways of interpreting world views as dictated by one's nervous system and the specific environment of our planetary existence."
Deepak Chopra[41]

You might be wondering how all this information applies to you? After all, not everyone reading this book will be experiencing their 'dark night of the soul', where life falls apart and you are given the chance to put it all back together with a new and enlightened sense of order and understanding.

It's all too common to hear people say, 'If I only had known then what I know now.' So, my invitation to you is: now that you *do* know more about the bigger picture, what would you like to do about it?

The first step to being able to bring about a change in your life and health is to understand how you view a situation. Not necessarily your conscious view, but, much more importantly, your deeper, subconscious view. You need to understand how you process information about that situation. It is not about how you control an event or how other people in your life feel about it; it is about how *you* feel. The aim is to arrive at this understanding before the stress of your situation becomes detrimental to your health; prevention is always better than cure.

---

41 'A Consciousness-based Science', Deepak Chopra MD, Menas Kafatos PhD and Rudolph H. Tanzi PhD, *Huffington Post*, New York, 11 September 2012.

Making the connections between life events, your thoughts about those events and the response of your body gives you the vital missing link that will help you to make changes to improve your health and happiness. This awareness changes the random symptoms of dis-ease into a valuable message from your body about your understanding of the world and of yourself.

Awareness of this connection goes only part of the way to resolving the issue, however. For deep and lasting change you will need to allow yourself to go deeper into the issue and to release the trauma held there, so that your perception can be updated and your body can regain its health. You will need to access your thoughts and understand what underlies them: your most basic perceptions and beliefs. To do this, you will need to understand something of how the mind works, how we store information and how we create the perceptions and beliefs with which we interpret our world.

Interpretation and response

We interpret the world around us metaphorically. That is, we translate what we see into something with which we are already familiar. (You might call a dysfunctional relationship with a partner 'a prison', for example.) However, while you may perceive the world in metaphors, your body is only able to respond literally. Let me give an example: if you feel in general that you are unable to set boundaries – in terms of your relationships, your job, or other people's expectations of you - your body will respond to your thinking by increasing the capacity in your bladder to hold more urine, with the purpose of enabling you literally to

> *The conscious mind is that part of the brain with which you plan, decide and compare. It is your awareness. Research has shown that we engage in conscious thinking on average only between two to five per cent of the time."*

better mark your territory (as a cat or dog does). While this is an amazingly intelligent mechanism, it is not altogether useful in modern society; social convention does not allow you to make such a literal gesture of boundary definition when challenged in the office or at home!

166

If the body has become engaged in responding to a problem in this literal way, then the issue is probably a deep one - even if you are not consciously aware of it. Imagine that you have not resolved an issue intellectually nor dealt with it on an emotional level. Then the body, acting on your behalf, will step in to make physical adaptations. In the example above, on a basic level your need to define your boundaries is considered a matter of your safety and survival, and the physical response supplied by your body is intended to resolve the situation.

The conscious mind

The conscious mind is that part of the brain with which you plan, decide and compare. It is your awareness. Research has shown that we engage in conscious thinking on average only between two to five per cent of the time. [42]

The conscious mind can process about 4,000 bits of information per second. This represents really focused thinking and requires concentration or application of thought. It is the part of the brain that applies willpower and positive thinking.

When you exercise your willpower or engage in positive thinking, you are using your conscious mind, because you have to concentrate upon your desired goal. This is why willpower is very difficult to apply - it requires such concentrated effort. I am sure you have experienced what it is like to tell yourself you should not do something, only to find that you do it anyway. In your conscious thinking, you are saying: 'No, I shouldn't have another chocolate', but there is another voice - a much more powerful one inside - that is saying, 'Yes, but you know you want to; it won't do any harm; it will make you feel better', 'One more won't hurt.' This quiet, persuasive and powerful inner voice is your subconscious mind.

---

42 'Mysteries of the Mind: Your Unconscious is Making Your Everyday Decisions', Marianne Szegedy-Maszak, *US News and World Report*, 20th February 2005, quoted by Bruce Lipton in *The Biology of Belief - Unleashing the Power of Consciousness, Matter & Miracles*, Bruce H. Lipton PhD, op. cit.

The subconscious mind

Our subconscious mind works to protect us. It works to keep us from re-experiencing the pain and trauma of past ordeals. This could be physical, mental or emotional pain.

It was Milton Erickson[43], an American psychiatrist and hypnotherapist and considered to be the grandfather of hypnotherapy, who said that, 'All problems were once solutions.'

What does this mean? Well, quite simply that the first time you did something to alleviate your pain or discomfort and it worked, your subconscious mind stored that information as a solution. This could be the chocolate that rewarded you and made you feel happier, the cigarette that calmed your nerves, the alcohol that made your forget the problem, and so on. To the subconscious mind, these are referenced as solutions to a given problem because they once worked. This is why willpower is so hard to apply in changing our behaviour while the subconscious mind has a different understanding and knows from experience that a desired result was achieved. The subconscious is often drawing on outdated information and applying it to the current situation.

There are distinct differences between the functions of the conscious mind and the subconscious mind. Compared with the conscious mind, the subconscious mind can process approximately 4,000,000,000 bits of information per second (that is, a million times faster) and requires no conscious effort upon your part at all.

Moreover, when the conscious mind is not actively engaged, the subconscious mind runs 95-98 per cent of your day-to-day thinking. Your subconscious mind is running constantly in the background. When you're concentrating with your conscious mind, it is still the subconscious that maintains your autonomic (automatic) bodily functions, your beliefs about who you are and your perception of the world. You're not consciously making your heart

---

43 *Seminars, Workshops and Lectures of Milton H. Erickson: Mind-body Communication in Hypnosis, in 3 volumes,* Milton H. Erickson, Free Association Books, London, 1998

beat, your blood pump or the muscles in your legs move when you walk, are you? Just imagine how complex an activity such as walking or talking would be if you had to consciously focus on each tiny movement, while also thinking about pumping your blood, balancing and breathing. These functions are fundamental tasks of your autonomic nervous system. Some of them are natural, like breathing, and some are learned and habitual, but begin to operate without your conscious thought, such as walking. Once you know how to perform these habitual tasks, the information is entered into your subconscious mind and you never forget it. Even if you do not walk for a while, you don't forget how to do it. Hence the expression, 'It's like riding a bike.'

Your beliefs operate in the same way. Once your subconscious mind has learned that 'the world is a dangerous place' or that 'people will misjudge me', these learned beliefs will be stored and run constantly in the background, as a reference by which you assess the world. The trouble is that, once we have formed a particular perception, we generalise the information. For example, if I assume that people will misjudge me and I noticed that my father pulled 'that face' when he did misjudge me, I now become sensitive to 'that face'. Anyone pulling 'that face' from now on could potentially misjudge me, so now this becomes a trigger for me to act in a particular way when I fear being misjudged.

You can imagine the subconscious mind operating like a powerful computer database and processor. It stores all the information you gather in case you need to reference it at any time. It's much like using a search engine.
Just like the internet, the capacity of the subconscious mind is vast. However, if you have ever used a search engine you will know that sometimes, when we enter a search, we get more than we bargained for. If someone has mislabelled their pages or pictures, or our search is not specific enough, we get curious results.

This is a bit like the way your subconscious mind works. Although you don't consciously realise it, every time you have any experience your subconscious mind captures everything that is present in your internal and external world at that point, for future reference. If your experience is a traumatic one, all this information is stored, but may be blanked from your conscious awareness

169

so that you are not consciously disturbed by the memory. However, all the specific and peripheral information around that event remains stored in your subconscious, so that you are equipped to avoid or to deal with a similar situation next time it occurs. This database of information is interconnected in the subconscious and there is no prioritising when it comes to referencing the information. Information in one column of the database is just as valid as data in another column.

Subconscious associations

Twelve-year-old Trevor is allergic to peanuts. They trigger his asthma. He has always been allergic to peanuts and it is assumed he has had the allergy from birth. Trevor was born prematurely and there were difficulties with his breathing when he was born, so he was whisked away from his mother and placed in a ventilator. This invasion of Trevor's breathing created a cerebral-cortex, territory-fear conflict (affecting the bronchial mucous membranes) and a territory fear 'can't cry out' (affecting the bronchial muscle). It transpired that throughout her pregnancy Trevor's mum had developed a craving for peanut butter and ate it constantly. Because the baby gets its supply of nutrients through the umbilical cord directly from its mother, peanuts were present in Trevor's system at the time of his birth. Trevor's subconscious took a snapshot of everything in his inner and outer world at the point of his traumatic birth, so that he could assess danger more easily next time he might encounter similar patterns. An association was made between the peanuts in his system and the traumatic event of his being taken away from his mother and having tubes put down his throat.

Now that he is older and encounters peanuts, Trevor's database cross-references the information that he stored at the time of his birth and makes a clear association with danger – a very specific danger – and the original bodily response to this danger is triggered. The bronchial mucous membranes are stimulated to compensate for an expected territorial invasion and the asthma symptoms begin.

The subconscious mind has no concept of time. To the subconscious mind, everything is happening in real time; everything is happening right now. This

> " *The subconscious mind has no concept of time. To the subconscious mind, everything is happening in real time; everything is happening right now.* "

is why the body responds immediately when you remember a threat or a previous traumatic event. The message that is sent instantaneously to the body is in the present, so the reaction is immediate. In this sense, the body does not know the difference between a real or an imagined threat. So re-living an event, or constantly referencing a painful memory or fearful thought, will send messages to the body to respond in exactly the same way as it would if the event were happening in the present moment.

Direct instruction

The subconscious mind prefers a direct instruction and cannot process negatives. It takes things literally. So when someone says 'Don't think of a pink elephant', the subconscious mind just hears, 'Think of a pink elephant.' You might want to think about this when giving simple instructions, especially to children. 'Don't knock that drink over' would be much better replaced with 'Be careful of the drink.' The child's subconscious mind is hearing 'Knock that drink over!' In the same way, the teacher who yells, 'Don't run in the corridor!' may get better results if she invites students to 'walk calmly in the corridor.'

How aware are you of your own thoughts? We all have conscious and subconscious thoughts. There are significant differences between the way your conscious and subconscious minds work, for important survival reasons. You act subconsciously without thinking. It is the default way in which you act, because it is based on your past experience. If you were told as a child that you could not have something, but found that if you stamped your feet and cried your parent would relent and give you what you wanted, this information was recorded in your subconscious mind as a successful behaviour.

However, although recorded behaviour can be useful, it can also create some undesirable effects if you are not aware. Using the example of the stamping child, imagine that if you do not get what you want today you would

171

automatically apply the same behaviour as your childhood default. Your response is deeply engrained in your subconscious mind as a working solution, but it is not a successful way of acting as an adult. So, we can say that specific events or aspects of a current situation, which you perceive to be the same as the early event, trigger you into this behaviour. To put it another way, aspects of your current situation are read by your subconscious mind, which instantly searches for how you succeeded in a similar, historic situation. Let us look at these reasons in detail now, starting with the concept of triggers.

How triggers work

A conscious trigger is something that reminds us of an event in such a way that we are aware of the connection between the thought and the earlier event. For example, a person who reminds you of a teacher who bullied you or an expression someone uses that takes you right back to the time your mother said the very same thing. Such conscious triggers will bring forth the very same responses that you experienced when you were in the original situation - the same physical sensations, thoughts and emotions. This can be difficult to handle if the trigger is a strong one and the event was deeply traumatic, but we can take steps to remedy the situation, provided we have an awareness of it.

Subconscious triggers are trickier to deal with, because we are not consciously aware of them. So, the first thing to do is to listen to your body, pay attention to your emotions and understand that something is happening under the surface. If you accept that the body does not make mistakes, it becomes possible to decode your response and find the trigger that has been recorded in the subconscious part of your mind.

Are you listening to your subconscious?

It may seem that listening to a somewhat childish inner voice is a far cry from the changes needed to make some improvements in your life. After all, you are likely to be confronted with difficult people every day, frustrating situations, pressures, and influences beyond your control. But it is how you meet those daily demands and, most importantly, how you perceive yourself in those situations that enables you, in a resourceful state, to cope or impacts on your health and wellbeing.

172

If you can start putting two and two together to understand your reactions, life will make a lot more sense. When you begin to listen to the messages and acknowledge the information that your body is giving you, you become the primary influence in your own life. Not only that, your life starts to change. Understanding what triggers you is like finding the key to the door of change.

Outdated beliefs

We each view the world through the belief filters that we construct as children. These filters are designed to keep us safe and to help us identify possible danger. However, sometimes these filters need cleaning out and renewing.

On a subconscious level, we still use those belief filters as a point of reference for our actions and behaviours. The beliefs and decisions you formed pre-six years' old have become the basis of your thoughts today. What appear to be rational thoughts and decisions on the surface may be built on a foundation of misunderstandings and the decisions of a frightened child. If you find that you are not happy with your life situation and with your health, perhaps it is time to dig down to examine the foundations of the structure.

I have learned to explain myself very clearly. I do this because of my early experiences in life when I felt misunderstood. More specifically, I felt misjudged. The experience of having someone close to me misjudge my motives had a great impact on me and, although I have done a lot of work on this issue, it is a very deep core belief that still surfaces at odd times. It is my 'Rome', to which all roads seem to lead.

Once you have formed your basic view of the world, your subconscious mind works very hard to prove that view correct. After all, you don't want to prove yourself wrong, do you? In order to preserve your belief system, the subconscious mind cleverly distorts information to fit your view, deletes information that doesn't fit, and generalises anything else that doesn't fit into a global picture. Your belief structure becomes cyclical.

I believe that I am misunderstood; it is a truth for me > I act as if it is true > I find evidence that it is true > the evidence confirms my belief.

173

For example, if you formed the belief when you were young that you are unlucky, you would notice every time you lost at a game, missed out on an opportunity, or didn't win a prize. And that would prove you right, of course. You would stop looking for the times you might win; you would stop spotting opportunities when you might gain something, because you would notice only what proves you right – the opportunity to lose. This process of self-reiteration occurs on many levels.

The way that we communicate is very interesting and fraught with possibilities for misunderstanding. We think we know what people mean, we think we know what 'that look' means, but really we are drawing on a great database of information stored in our own subconscious mind. When we perceive something, we are referencing what we already know in order to make sense of what we are now experiencing. This process either reiterates what we already believe or adds new information.

Updating the database
Changing your thoughts about and reactions to a situation is different to managing your thoughts and reactions in the face of an event.

It is possible to manage stressful thoughts and situations. Most stress coaches teach you ways in which to change your state, such as breathing techniques or visualisation, in order to bring you out of stress. However, following the two phases of an illness, as discussed in Chapter 4, the subconscious mind has already triggered the stress message to the body (phase one), so the body must still go through a process of resolution and regeneration (phase two) to resolve the triggered response. This means that you can still experience symptoms when you enter the second phase of rest and repair, even if that happens almost immediately after you were initially triggered into stress.

For example, when Graham's younger brother came along, Graham missed sitting on his mother's knee as he used to. He felt he had lost that intimate contact with his mother, because she was too busy with the baby. At this point, the skin on the back of Graham's legs and lower back, where he had had contact with his mother, became thin and desensitised so that Graham would not miss the physical contact with his mother so much. Graham's mum would still occasionally call him to sit on her knee and this would afford him some comfort. When this happened, however, Graham would enter into the second phase and his skin would begin to repair – showing the symptoms of eczema. Even if Graham constantly reminded himself that he would still have some contact with his mother, seeing her with the baby kept triggering him to miss the contact and the way things used to be. He experienced resolution when he could again sit on her lap, and he also became more used to her not having time for him, but he still missed the way in which they used to be closer. Despite resolving the loss of contact in a number of ways, therefore, Graham was still triggered into stress by being reminded that he had lost that intimate contact.

This is why people who meditate and manage their stress still seem to encounter health problems. No matter how well you 'manage' your stress, your body will still pass through the two phases of dis-ease, unless - and this is crucial - you actually 'release' the triggers that cause your stressful reactions. To release, or emotionally to come to terms with the original event, means that you will no longer be triggered into the die-ease process.

Revisiting memories

Your memories change every time you look at them. This is because *you* have changed every time you look at them. Every time you look at a memory, you are a different person and cannot possibly have the very same perspective that you had at any other time. When you revisit a memory, there will be aspects that were strong at the time that memory was recorded. These aspects grow stronger every time you look at the memory and become more exaggerated as the neural pathways in your brain grow stronger with repetition. At the same time, the information that you do not revisit begins to fade. This means that all of your memories are distortions of the truth. And anyway, the truth as you saw it was merely a perspective that you formed at that time.

The more you repeat a thought, the more you strengthen the neural pathways and synapses in the brain which carry that thought, making the connections quicker next time. This means that when you learn something and as you become more familiar with it, you change the cellular structure of your brain. Connections that are not made often weaken. This ability of the brain to change its structure through learning is called neuroplasticity. This process also occurs when you think the same thought often or frequently revisit a past memory. The connections to a specific way of thinking become stronger and easier to use, whereas the connections to less-used thoughts become weaker and eventually redundant.

This is interesting, if you think about that fact, that our memories are a distortion of reality to begin with. If we access a memory on a regular basis, it can become increasingly distorted in its importance.

How triggers affect the dis-ease process

Habitual thinking and limiting beliefs are as effective as ongoing, actual danger in triggering the body and keeping it trapped in a dis-ease cycle.

James had ongoing rhinitis[44]. When we discussed his symptoms in order to identify the root cause, it became clear from his phrasing how he was manifesting the illness.

We know that the symptoms of rhinitis occur in the second phase of the two phases of dis-ease, when the nasal lining or mucous membranes is regenerating after the stress has passed. In order to locate the turning point from stress to regeneration, I asked James what annoying situation he had felt better about just before the last bout started. He was able to bring to mind a person who had been annoying him at work and from this we could also identify his patterns of thought.

James is a placid and gentle soul and when I asked him how he handled this annoying person, he said, 'Well, I just tell myself, "You're never going to be able to change some people, so you may as well let it go".' This statement reveals why James continues to have ongoing symptoms of rhinitis. He does not spend a lot of time in stress because he quickly resolves the issue and accepts the situation. However, he is still triggered into annoyance in the first

---

44 Rhinitis is a medical term for irritation and inflammation of the mucous membrane inside the nose. Common symptoms of rhinitis are a stuffy nose, runny nose, and post-nasal drip. Wikipedia

place, so quickly enters into the repair phase and experiences the symptoms of rhinitis. Without addressing the issue that triggers him, he will continue to go through this cycle of trigger-stress-resolution-repair over and over again. If he is already in the process of healing one annoyance and is triggered again by a new one, his symptoms will get even worse, not better.

Habitual thinking and limiting beliefs are as effective as ongoing, actual danger in triggering the body and keeping it trapped in a dis-ease cycle."

Consciously, James is aware that he cannot change other people and doesn't think he should try. He can bring himself to accept their behaviour and is then able to let go of the situation. However, he still seems to be triggered initially into annoyance at their behaviour. There is a deeper trigger at work somewhere in his subconscious mind. Something about their behaviour subconsciously reminds him of an earlier time, when he was annoyed at a similar behaviour. He was not really aware that he was especially annoyed until he examined the situation more closely.

If you think about that fact, that our memories are a distortion of reality to begin with. If we access a memory on a regular basis, it can become increasingly distorted in its importance."

177

A number of different outcomes were possible for James:

- He could have been annoyed with the person, come to terms with the situation and moved through the two phases without being re-triggered. He would have had one instance of a cold.
- He could have been annoyed and come to terms with the issue and moved through the two phases, and then encountered the problem again and experienced a fresh annoyance, taking him through the cycle again.
- He could have been annoyed and kept thinking of how annoying the situation was, thus continuing to re-trigger the stress and staying in the stress phase, although he would not get any symptoms while the nasal mucous membranes thinned. His breathing would be fine until he resolved the situation, but then he would enter a lengthy period of symptom-laden repair.
- Finally, he could have been annoyed, felt better about the issue, but kept dwelling on the situation and thinking about the annoying situation. This is what had actually happened in James's case.

Using some simple memory-recall techniques, James was able to make the connection between this recurring illness and an original event, when he had formed a belief around a related issue. The trigger was something he heard, saw, felt or even smelled or tasted and which brought forth the original memory. The person who had annoyed him recently had copied the design of his website. This reminded him of a time at school when his best friend had copied his work, despite his having said that he couldn't, and they had both got into trouble. He had been unable to stop his friend's behaviour, so felt he had to 'be the better person' and endure or ignore the incident, but it had still annoyed him. He had formed the belief – which he still holds - that 'people are lazy'. This is the underlying reason that he was unable to let the issue go – and why it still acted as a trigger for his annoyance in similar situations.

Are you responding to triggers?

Your triggers don't have to be big to be effective. They can be very simple but deeply rooted beliefs, which were formed at a time when you needed to understand the way the world operated in order to function appropriately. We all have our 'elephants in the room' and sometimes they are clear to us, but at other times they are hidden under layers and patterns of thinking. I often find that the more intelligent the person, the more complex their network of thoughts and the more devious their techniques to avoid getting to the core of the issue. After all, your belief is not a belief – it's true, right? Your beliefs are as real to you as the air you breathe and the sun that sets in the morning. You see your beliefs as facts.

Try this exercise.

1. Make a list of ten negative facts you know to be true about yourself or your life. Try to choose things that affect your emotions, such as:

    •   My spouse does not listen to me
    •   I cannot lose weight
    •   I am terrible in the mornings.

2. For each item, rate out of 100 per cent how true this fact is for you.

3. For each item, write three different times you have seen clear evidence of this truth, for example 'When I told my husband about what my boss said, he didn't pay proper attention, he only grunted and continued to read his paper.'

4. Now for each item, write three different pieces of evidence that this is *not* true. For example, the times it didn't happen or you know differently.

5. Read through your list and re-grade out of 100 per cent how true each item now seems to be, in the light of the possible evidence that these 'facts' are *not* true.

This is a simple exercise, to draw your attention to how easily we delete, distort or generalise things without realising it. We turn our thoughts and beliefs into 'facts', when actually they are simply our own perspectives. With this in mind, it is a good idea to start observing your own thoughts and beliefs. Are they serving you or are they now at the root of your illnesses or limited life situations?

Reading the signposts

You might not be as in control of your thoughts as you think. How would you know if you weren't? We tend to go about our daily business only really aware of our conscious thoughts - and some of us might not even be aware of those. We don't like to admit that we are not in control of our thoughts. It doesn't feel right to admit that we do not have full control of how we act and respond. However, the conscious mind can do only so much, so we are mostly responding and reacting with the information stored in our subconscious mind, even if that doesn't chime with what we consciously want in life.

One good way to observe what your subconscious thoughts are about a situation is to listen to what we call 'tail-enders'. By tail-enders, I mean the trailing afterthoughts that accompany our conscious thoughts. If you have ever tried 'affirmations' or using your willpower to change your habits, you might be familiar with the trailing after-comments that follow your positive statements. An example would be when you affirm 'I am worthy of love' and then hear an inner voice saying, 'That's rubbish!; Who says?; What, me?; Yeah, right!' or any number of personal rebukes.

Tail-enders are clues to the subconscious argument that goes on in the background - the part of your thinking that you try to ignore when you're applying your willpower. When you have a conscious thought, your tail-enders, or 'yes, buts' as they are often called, can give you much more information than you realise. It does not have to be a voice in your head, it can be a feeling or sensation in your body. It is something that makes you aware that 'This is not true for me.'

Try this simple experiment. Take a deep breath, say each of the following statements out loud and wait for your inner response. Make a note of the tail-enders - the feelings and sensations or voice in your head. It may begin with a positive response that trails off into a 'yes, but' or an 'except...'. Do it a few times, until you are used to listening to that inner voice or feeling.

- I am a beautiful person
- I deserve a million pounds
- I will be fully healthy.

What did your subconscious tell you? Your inner voice may seem insignificant, or even random. It is very personal to you and may point the way to deeper beliefs.

I tried these statements three times and my personal responses to each of these statements were quite mixed. I also had different issues that came up at different times. This in itself is very interesting and might mean I am accessing different past situations as points of reference. Because I am quite visual, as well as my inner voice I also visualised pictures. Some of my tail-enders were as follows:

- *I am a beautiful person*
  - So I shouldn't get angry (which I still sometimes do, so I cannot be a beautiful person, because beautiful people don't get angry).
  - But I'd be selfish if I said 'no' to people (to be beautiful and good, nice people don't say 'no' to doing things for other people, so if I do say 'no', I am not a nice person).
  - I shouldn't make mistakes (which I do, so therefore I am not beautiful).
  - I also had an image - a memory of me hitting my partner when I was in a very badly drunken, angry state. This image tells me: 'No, I am not a beautiful person - I am a bad person.'

181

- *I deserve a million pounds*
  - ○ I haven't earned a million pounds
  - ○ It would be selfish to have a million pounds
  - ○ People won't like me if I have a million pounds
  - ○ I also had a physical, agitated feeling in my tummy and in my knees, as if I wanted to run away.

- *I can be totally healthy*
  - ○ You will never have enough energy
  - ○ You're always tired in the morning
  - ○ It's hard work to stay healthy
  - ○ I also had a feeling of tiredness and of being overwhelmed, which is the feeling I get when I have taken too much on and feel I cannot keep up.

I consciously agree with all three of these statements: I am a beautiful person - we all are; I do deserve a million pounds; and I can be totally healthy. I believe that I am healthy and, yet, my subconscious mind seems to have a different idea. It is this mind that is in charge of my thinking for 95-98 per cent of the time. And this part of my brain is far more powerful than my conscious mind.

Try the exercise again with something that is especially relevant to you. For example:

- I will meet the right person and be happy
- I will give up chocolate/smoking/biting my nails
- [Something relevant to your personal circumstances at the moment].

If you have heard of the Law of Attraction[45] (what you think about, you can manifest in your life) and wonder how or why it works, it is worth bearing in mind that we attract life experiences through our subconscious thoughts, not our conscious thoughts. Positive thinking does not necessarily change your circumstances on its own, especially if you constantly try to think positively, but elicit the tail-ender (counter-argument) from your subconscious. It is necessary to go beneath it and to accept that there is an internal battle going on. Dig to find the root of it.

What are your priorities?

We all have priorities in life. What matters most to you on a day-to-day basis? Do you have goals and dreams? Or, like many, are you just struggling to get through the day? Do you desire a better relationship, a better home life, a better job, more time with loved ones, more time to yourself or better health?

Now might be a good time to look at what really matters in your life so that you can begin to examine what strains are preventing you from achieving it. It is never about other people, although it might seem so. *It is always about your own thoughts and beliefs and the way in which you create the world around you.* This doesn't mean to say that someone else's behaviour should be tolerated if it is undesirable or unhealthy for you, but the responsibility to do what is healthy for *you* falls on *you*. If you cannot change a situation, changing the way you *feel* about it is far healthier than enduring or resisting it.

Your personal experiences

What would it mean to you to be in control of your subconscious thoughts and beliefs? First, you will need to accept that they exist and to appreciate them for what they are - a fundamental survival mechanism. It may be true now that your early beliefs are limiting your success in some areas of your life, or even causing dis-ease in your body. Without acknowledging their initial purpose was to protect you, judgment or denial will only compound the problem.

---

45 See, for example, *Think and Grow Rich*, Napoleon Hill, Fawcett Books, New York, 1960

Remember how incredible your body is and how exquisitely organised and structured it is. Your body has known how to respond and adapt to threat or danger very precisely. Your amazing body has adapted and changed with the express intention to function better under strain. And your innate survival skills have enabled you to download information and programmes at a very early age so that you would be safe to survive in the world.

So what is the problem? The primary problem is that we are social animals operating under constraints and social boundaries, unlike animals in the wild that are not prevented by convention from reacting. We do not process and release our traumatic experiences naturally as an animal in the wild would release the freeze response. Instead, we store trauma in the body. A trauma does not have to be a momentous, violent or life-threatening trauma. When you are young, it can be a simple misunderstanding or mis-perception. Something like being ignored by a parent, being forgotten, or not allowed to join in could all be perceived as threats to survival when you are young. As you grow older, you adjust to different contexts and life situations, but you still reference the early lessons that were hard-wired into your subconscious mind during your formative years.

> *However, if you listen to your subconscious, however irrational it may seem, you can discover your greatest blockages to health, wealth and success.* "

The more traumas and stressful life events you experience, the more strain is put upon your body. No matter how you consciously choose to live your life, your daily routine will throw up reminders and 'triggers' that will constantly reference your early beliefs. This creates a constant battle between the conscious mind and the subconscious mind and your body and health can be compromised by the cross-currents created from this tension.

Whether we realise it or not, we are driven to resolve our own early traumas and perceptions. For me, this was the fear of not being understood, the fear of being misjudged. It has guided my life choices and driven me to where I am now.

Your personal events and traumas

Admitting that you have powerful subconscious thoughts is not easy. Especially as the subconscious mind is very child-like and the language that it uses is equally child-like. Most people rationalise their thoughts and tell themselves 'not to be so silly'. However, if you listen to your subconscious, however irrational it may seem, you can discover your greatest blockages to health, wealth and success.

Let us take again my example of fearing that people will misjudge me.

The process of thought is as follows:

- People will misunderstand me. This means ...
- they will misjudge me. This means ...
- they will think badly of me. This means ...
- they will think I am a bad person. This means ...
- they will not like me. This means ...
- I cannot be myself. This means ...
- I can't do what I want to do in life. This means ...
- I cannot fulfil my purpose in life.

And if we take this even further, not being able to be myself and fulfil my purpose in life means I may as well not bother: I am helpless and life is hopeless. In fact, it becomes a survival issue.

My thoughts are not unusual or different those of most people; it just takes time to listen to the child-like thoughts of the subconscious mind, so that we may make the connections to what matters to us. Listening and really hearing what is going on underneath opens up the world of change to us. Our limiting beliefs are holding us back and are based on outdated information. These beliefs are the product of decisions made from experiences faced at much earlier stages in our life and, although they are no longer true or even

185

helpful in our current situations, they are still the decisions and beliefs by which we operate.

Acknowledging that there is a programme running

It is possible to track back to the root cause of a specific symptom, by using the time frame of its last appearance. However, finding the core beliefs that underpin and link multiple symptoms or repeated manifestations is crucial to unravelling the way in which an illness becomes all-pervading. Those core beliefs may not consciously make any sense. It is only by delving into the subconscious mind that you will be able to see how the belief system that you are operating with gives you information to act and respond in the world. You may have a conscious thought or desire, but your way of really being in the world will be driven by your subconscious beliefs, and you will draw conclusions and make decisions based on those beliefs. Your body acknowledges these conclusions with the required response - after all, your body is merely an extension of your thoughts and beliefs. There is no separation between body and mind.

9. Your lifestyle is your health

"Once social change begins, it cannot be reversed. You cannot uneducate the person who has learned to read. You cannot humiliate the person who feels pride. You cannot oppress the people who are not afraid anymore."
Cesar Chavez[46]

I f you really start to grasp the significance and the implications of the META-Health approach, you might like to start thinking about how these principles can be applied more widely. How is your health affected by your familial, social and work situations? How can this information contribute to resolving family and relationship problems, or wellness and wellbeing at work?

When you understand the difference between the conscious and subconscious mind, it's possible to realise that, although you might consciously want one thing, you may be manifesting something quite different that is based on your subconscious beliefs. You might strive for a loving relationship, but if you do not believe that you deserve or will ever achieve one, your behaviour will result in you fulfilling your subconscious beliefs instead of your conscious ones. The conflicts arising from this incongruity can result in ill health.

To be able to assess whether you are creating your reality as you would wish it to be, you have to consider how you react in the different aspects of your life. Are your needs being met at home, in relationships, in your work?

Health is about balance. If your needs are not being met in some important areas of your life, the stress of trying to compensate may cause ill health. It

---

46 Cesar Chavez, Founder and President of the United Farm Workers of America, AFL-CIO, 'Address to The Commonwealth Club of California', 9 November 1984, San Francisco, USA

is not enough to manage your stressors. A healthy lifestyle is a lifestyle where inner conflicts are at a minimum or at the very least, dealt with, processed and released, rather than pushed down and embodied.

With this framework of understanding, it is possible to gain a fuller 'META' perspective - not just on your health, but on your lifestyle. If you see all aspects of your life as either contributing to or draining your health and happiness, you might want to reassess where you are focusing your energy and what impact that is having on your health.

There is a body-mind-social connection

There have been numerous studies about the effects of meditation on groups of people. One of the most famous is the study in 1993 of a group of 4,000 people collectively sitting in transcendental meditation in Washington DC[47]. The study showed that, during the one-month period during which participants were meditating collectively, the rate of violent crime (as measured by police statistics) dropped significantly (by 23 per cent) and continued to decrease as the number of people meditating increased. It was predicted that if the group continued at the same rate, the serious crime rate would drop by 48 per cent. With each individual simply holding a calm and centred space, the behaviour and responses of people outside that space was affected. How might this apply to you in your family and social situations? How does your energy affect those around you?

Biological, psychological and social health

The ten META principles provide a framework for health. This is not just physical health, but extends to psychological and social health. Indeed, it is not really possible to draw a distinction between personal and social health, since our interaction with each other as social beings is fundamental to our own individual health and wellbeing.

---

47 'Effects of Group Practice of the *Transcendental Meditation* Program on Preventing Violent Crime in Washington, D.C.: Results of the National Demonstration Project, June–July 1993', John S. Hagelin, Maxwell V. Rainforth, David W. Orme-Johnson, Kenneth L. Cavanaugh, Charles N. Alexander, Susan F. Shatkin, John L. Davies, Anne O. Hughes and Emanuel Ross, *Social Indicators Research*, **47**: 153-201, Kluwer Academic Publishers, Amsterdam, 1999

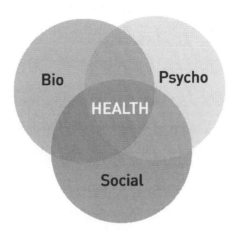

Fig.13 The biological, psychological, social connection

You might think that your beliefs are your own, but you learned them from your parents and other influences in the very earliest years of your life. Through observation and instruction, you adopted your preferred way to be in the world from the people who were close to you as you grew up.

We have evolved as social animals and depend on our social bond to create balance and harmony. Society is an extension of personal health and our personal health is a reflection of our social health.

The more we release our own traumas and are able to respond meaningfully rather than simply react to situations, the more we affect other people and we affect those situations. We all create our own worlds around us, the drama queen attracts and creates drama, a hippy has love and peace, man! What kind of reflection do you have of how you are in your world?

Beliefs are catching

You share perspectives and beliefs. You share your views of the world with your family, your friends and work colleagues. You share societal and cultural views and form opinions based on the views of the media you select.

You might think that your beliefs are your own, but you learned them from your parents and other influences in the very earliest years of your life. Through observation and instruction, you adopted your preferred way to be in the world from the people who were close to you as you grew up. But your learning does not stop there. As you ventured into new social situations you learned from those around you how to think and to act in the world. Teachers and organisations create rules that you adopt and, as you conform to convention, you in turn teach those conventions to others.

Living in the world you create

We might not like the idea, but we do live in a world that we create for ourselves. I can say that it has taken some time for me to develop this perspective. Before I understood how powerful my thoughts and beliefs were in manifesting my health, wealth and happiness, I would have scoffed at such an idea. When you are in the midst of suffering, it is very difficult to take the higher perspective from which change can occur.

Understanding physical and psychological illness from the META perspective at least gives you the ladder with which to climb to that higher perspective. The META-Health principles are the rungs on the ladder and, from that height, you can view afresh the situations in which you find yourself. You can take a more resourceful view of your emotions, responses, actions and behaviours. If you are able to be the observer of your own physical symptoms and emotional responses, you will be able to have a significant impact on your personal health.

It is not about whether you act or not in a situation; it is about choosing to act from a position of calm. It may still be necessary to speak your mind, to reprimand someone or to express displeasure. It may be the appropriate response. However, being overwhelmed by anger, or any other emotion, may result in actions beyond your control that will not produce your desired outcome. Moreover, if we look at the bigger picture, we have a responsibility not only to ourselves, but to other people with whom we engage. An assertive person looks for the 'win/win' outcome without aggression and without conceding to unreasonable demands. The aggressive person is interested only in winning, while the passive person is able only to concede.

Think of this when you consider different contexts of your life. Are you assertive in your home life, with your family? Are you assertive at work, with colleagues and bosses? If you start to peel away the layers of the onion of assertiveness, you will find that there are many layers, leading to a central core of self-worth.

The human spectrum

One of the greatest gifts that the META perspective has given me is to understand what other people have been through in their lives. I find that when I see people in the street, people with certain illnesses or behaving in a certain way, I feel more patience and compassion.

Everyone is different and, although we have basic human needs, the way we perceive and meet those needs is very individual. What to one person is important, to another may be insignificant. Language and communication also serve to bring an added dimension of confusion to life. We each think that we are the only one who sees reality in the way it really is, but we each have our own version of reality. Innocent statements and actions can be read quite differently, depending on your personal interpretation. Such interpretations are based on the core beliefs that were formed at a young age.

I had an interesting realisation just recently, when talking to my husband about what we would cook for dinner. We are vegetarians and were selecting a combination of vegetables that would make a nice meal. We both cook, but Vic has been taking on a lot more of the cooking while I have been writing this book. We selected a range of veg and Vic asked if I wanted anything else, perhaps also some carrots? I said, 'No thanks, I think we have plenty here,' to which Vic replied, 'Are you sure?'

Now, this is an ordinary enough conversation, but based on our different backgrounds and beliefs, two different things were being said here. If we think about the core beliefs that we both have, we can see how our individual interpretations become part of the conversation.

Vic has the belief that everything is his responsibility, that *everything that goes wrong is his fault* and he has to make everything right. He is ever-vigilant in order not to upset people and so felt the need to double-check that I was sure, because he did not want a situation later in which I was still hungry and did not have enough food. He would have felt that it was his fault that he had not cooked enough, that he had let me down and that I would be upset because of something he had 'got wrong'.

When Vic asked me if I was sure, I heard 'I don't believe you', because of course my core belief is that people will misunderstand me, misjudge me or not believe me. I had given him an answer and he was not accepting it; he must think I am not really sure of what I want or I am not telling the truth; he could of course want me to change my mind, which may mean he does not respect or validate my decisions. Understanding the different core beliefs we were coming from made it possible for us to avoid a conflict over carrots! This is only a tiny and slightly comical example, but this sort of thing happens all the time between couples. The trick is to take ownership of your part of the interaction. If you are looking for a win/win situation, there is no conflict in taking ownership of your own reaction and accepting it for what it is. Better that we love the other people in our life for being where they are at and doing their best, than feeling that everything they say and do is about us.

Cause and effect on a bigger scale
When we begin to take ownership of our thoughts and triggers, it becomes possible to see the impact that our actions have on those around us.

You have an influence on all the people you meet in daily life. It begins with the way you interact with your family and extends to your friends, colleagues and even to strangers you pass in the street. One of the most amazing gifts I have found from understanding the META-Heath principles is the understanding it gives me of other people. I have always tried to be patient and thoughtful – not always easy when something is not going your way or someone is being particularly unpleasant or difficult. However, the META perspective has granted me a new dimension to my understanding, giving me the ability to take things less personally. Because the META-Health understanding extends way beyond the root cause of mere physical symptoms and into explaining psychological behaviour, I am more readily aware of my reactions to other people. This is because I can see their behaviour for what it is – an adaptation to manage the situation. Therefore, it's not about me – although *my reaction* is about me!

Imagine taking this understanding into different aspects of your life. It could help you understand the dynamics of your family better, or the personal issues of people at work that drove them to behave in certain ways. Do you think it would help you to disengage from what could be upsetting situations and potential triggers for stress and illness? It works both ways - I use this understanding to spot my own triggers and thoughts, so that I can deal with and process them instead of creating stress and possible illness in myself. But I can also spot other people's triggers and behaviours. This gives a fresh perspective on how we all interact socially and how confusions, selfishness and fear creep into our daily social situations. When fear is a part of the equation, we exhibit reactions that appear to be a much more selfish and animalistic response.

Fear triggers our primal and early survival programmes. Transcending fear is not easy if we do not see it in its proper place and for what it is.

Family dynamics

If you imagine your energy as a droplet in a pool of water, the ripples flow outwards and meet with ripples from other droplets. Once started, the ripples can reach far and wide and keep going. You make those ripples at home, at work and with everyone with whom you come into contact. You spread your ripples out into the world, even without realising you are doing so. Just as you receive the ripples that other people send out, your ripples may trigger someone else, either intentionally or unintentionally. All you can do is to be aware of your intentions and what triggers you when going about your daily business. Then, if you are triggered yourself, you can be aware of how that makes you respond.

Feeling wronged creates great energy in some people and can be the beginning of a long relationship of negative thoughts and behaviours, leading to ill health. If you feel wronged, what lies beneath that thought? If you set out to hurt another person, it is likely to evoke an equally negative response. It is not a win/win scenario. If you feel the need to be mean or harmful to another person, I suggest you look at why you feel that way. What justification do you give yourself for that feeling – where does that belief come from? Why do you take that person's actions so personally that you can respond in such a way? What is going on inside *you* that bestows such power on the other person to upset you?

The most difficult emotion to let go of is anger. Most people feel they have great justification for displaying anger; it is a great motivator. Also, letting go of anger for some people is like saying that what happened is OK. People cannot differentiate between accepting that something happened and letting it go and showing acceptance of what happened. Only when you have truly accepted that what happened did happen will it become possible to see that anger only corrodes the angered party. As the Buddha said: 'Holding on to anger is like grasping a hot coal with the intent of throwing it at someone else; you are the one who gets burned.'

You are your parents' child

Feeling wronged by a specific action or attitude may be something you learned from your parents. I find it both terrifying and hilarious that I become my mother when I am upset. I see my face, my waving finger, and hear the exact words, in the same tone and inflection as my mother. I am triggered by very similar things to those that triggered my mother and, even though I am aware of duplicating her response, it still rises as a reaction from my subconscious mind. There are two possible reasons for this and they fall into the 'nature' and 'nurture' categories. This argument has been going on for centuries, but in my opinion there is no conflict in accepting both interpretations.

You inherit thoughts and beliefs from your parents even in the womb. Both physiologically *and* energetically you are a combination of your mother and father, so how could you not inherit some of their energetic make-up?
You are also in the womb for nine months, receiving all the energetic and chemical messages flying around your mother's body and, at some point, you

194

begin to hear and to sense the outer world while still in the womb. By the time you are born into the world, you already possess your first beliefs and programmes about how to function in the world. This is further extended by your learning path in your early years.

How do you know what is your own belief and what is an inherited one? Well, basically, you don't. Whether you inherited it in your energetic system or in your genes, or whether you learned it from your parents or carers pre-six years' old, you were equipped with a system of beliefs when you went out into the world that determines how you perceive and how you respond to others. You consider these beliefs to be the truth about how the world is and you consider them to be absolute. However, if they are beliefs based on inherited information or on perceptions that arise from a particular viewpoint, do they really have to be set in stone? The problem is that once they are inside your subconscious, it is difficult to access them from 'outside the box'. This is because, working from your own perspective, you are already working 'inside the box' created by those beliefs.

Take, for example, the concept of land and territory. The idea that your country should be defended at the price of your own life if necessary is a strong truth for many people. It is so strong that young men and women are ready to participate in wars by signing up to 'fight for peace'. But is this idea 'true'? Is it true that the other party will take over and take what is yours? We usually see in others what we feel in ourselves. (The person that has been unfaithful lives in fear of their partner being unfaithful.) As already discussed, we look for evidence of the truth that we believe and do not look beyond it. We hold our beliefs to be the truth for everyone else too; yet, the more people change their beliefs - and in the case of war, they are beliefs based on fear - the more we can change the wider human consciousness. It is hard to see fear from the inside. When you are afraid you are not enough in yourself, you become afraid that you do not have enough, and that there will not be enough. You become open to the fear that someone else will take what is yours. To compensate for that fear, you take more and so the belief continues its cycle. Because you take more, others have less and everyone becomes afraid of not having enough. The consumer society is based on the fear that 'I am not enough' or 'I am not good enough', so that it is only by having and consuming that we can feel good about ourselves. We are taught from an early age that we must fit in with this scheme. So, our physical manifestations of dis-ease are sown along with those early beliefs.

Repeating patterns

When we pass on those beliefs, we perpetuate the same patterns that created the dis-ease. If you have a dis-ease running in your family, you may be convinced it's a genetic problem, but you can be sure that there will be a common belief system underlying it, which will hold the dis-ease in place. Are you aware that you can break the cycle? It is possible for you to uncover the beliefs that hold your illness in place, even if it is one that has been passed down your family line. Using META-Health to uncover the root cause makes it possible to clear the triggers that are creating the loop that perpetuates the illness. META-Health can free you from passing on those illnesses.

Pushing all the right buttons

Someone 'pushes my buttons' is such a great expression. It is the perfect metaphor for what happens to you when you are triggered by something. The button is pushed and the reaction takes place. Because it is a subconscious response, it usually happens beyond your control and before you know it. The feeling is already present. The bio-logical response is already activated. I once heard Ram Dass say, 'So you think you are a spiritual person? Go visit your family.' It is interesting that some of our most challenging triggers can come from those nearest and dearest to us. If each small trauma that you experienced as you were growing up was stored in your subconscious, is it any wonder that the people who were present when you formed your decisions about yourself and the world are the perfect triggers to remind you exactly of those past times? On the surface, you are grown up and have moved on, but when your mother or father says something or looks at you in that 'certain way', you are instantly transported by your subconscious mind back to the time when you were hurt or traumatised as a child by a similar comment or look. The specific meaning that you assigned to that comment or look at the time of the trauma is what that comment or look means to you now. Not only that, but your feelings and behaviour will be those of the childish you who suffered the original hurt, rather than the grown-up you. It doesn't matter how old or grown-up you are now, your response is that of the child who was hurt. And, of course, if you act and respond in this way, it sets the stage for the same behaviour all round as everyone slips back into their old patterns.

The ecology of change

Change is difficult. I urge you to begin to notice your behaviour and your responses and to begin to see the impact your thoughts have on your health.

> *I once heard Ram Dass say, 'So you think you are a spiritual person? Go visit your family.' It is interesting that some of our most challenging triggers can come from those nearest and dearest to us."*

I also urge you to notice how you will begin to change the world around you by disengaging from the same old patterns and responses towards other people. This change in your steps of the dance you are doing together can of course be a little scary for the other people involved!

When you begin to change and no longer engage in the same patterns of behaviour, people are forced to become aware of their own behaviours. If you choose not to respond with anger, but you merely notice that something your partner has said triggered you, their anger will not fuelled. Although it may take time, patterns of response will change for both of you.

If you do not mirror the behaviour directed at you, you become a mirror that merely reflects back the other person's behaviour.

You are probably reading this book because you want to make changes. But be aware that some people do not want to change and that trying to change someone else is most likely to result in frustration and disappointment. You can lead only by example, or to quote the saying often ascribed to Gandhi, 'Be the change that you want to see in the world.' Be prepared for some resistance from those around you who feel that they know you and are used to you the way that you have always been. It is a good idea to be accepting of their limitations while you explore the parts of your life that are affecting your health and the things that support your positive and active return to health.

People can easily be thrown when someone shifts from a previous, predictable behaviour into a new pattern of behaviour. It means that their world too has to change - and change can be frightening. It is much better to lead those around you into gentle change than it is to create a whirlwind around people and leave them bewildered and on the defensive. Men and women respond differently to change and to discussion, this is worth bearing in mind'.

Friendship and social groups

Once you know what your key stressors are, and how your beliefs interact with your triggers, it's possible to observe how and when this happens. I usually ask clients to keep a simple diary of when they notice their symptoms changing, also noting when their mood, behaviour and circumstances change. People usually spend time with those with whom they resonate best. They either share common interests, views or circumstances. If you have an illness that has become part of your lifestyle, for example, it can be very difficult to change your patterns when this may mean rocking the boat and affecting your social groups and friendships.

Are you picking up good vibrations from the people around you? We resonate with what we hold and believe, so I wonder if you are resonating with healthy, life-affirming beliefs or whether, at the moment, you are drawn to people who hold the same limiting beliefs as you, people who are also helping to hold your dis-ease in place by reinforcement?

A really common example of this is weight-loss groups. Imagine that you are desperate to lose weight and have made best friends with the people in your weight-loss group. Once you have reached your target weight, you will no longer need the weight-loss group and therefore may lose your friends who understand you so well. In your conscious mind, you are desperate to become slimmer, but there may be a subconscious resistance because of the consequences of what might happen if you do lose the weight - losing your friends too!

This kind of response can happen in any situation. A wife who had chronic fatigue (possible beliefs: 'I am not good enough'; 'I need to be perfect'; 'the world is a dangerous place') was well supported by her husband when she became ill. He had not paid her any attention before, but now she was ill he was loving and attentive. She wanted to get well, but feared he would lose interest in her again if she did.

A child with asthma (fear of someone entering or leaving your territory beyond your control) got more attention from his mother than his siblings when he had difficulty breathing. He feared that if he were to recover fully, he would not get her full and undivided attention any more.

Change is difficult and it is necessary to delve beneath the presenting behaviour and symptoms in order to understand what can be done on a deeper level to heal earlier traumas, which define how you feel and act in the world today. Take a look at your world afresh. Where do things and people around you reflect your own beliefs back to you? What do you see in your friends that you have not been noticing in yourself?

Imagine that your friends are a mirror of who you are. All that you like and dislike about them can be a reflection of what you see in the world - and what we see in the world is what we hold inside. So, take a good look and see yourself with fresh eyes. What is it that you praise in your friends that perhaps you should be noticing and praising in yourself? It's really easy to be kind to others and to appreciate their qualities - much easier than praising yourself. Alternatively, what is it about your friends that annoys you? Is it possible that these traits are something that you yourself need to address? When you become the observer of your thoughts and behaviour, it is possible to see what an impact you already have on your own health and happiness. With the right tools, you become aware how much impact you *can* have in the world.

Children especially pick up on emotions and energy, from parents, teachers and friends. However much you might try to hide your thoughts and feelings from others, your energetic presence gives it away. Our basic instinct is to read other people's energies in order to know how to respond and react; therefore, if you are not congruent with your energy you will send mixed and confusing signals.

The honesty of not knowing

I have a very strong belief that children should not be lied to. Children are very intuitive and pick up on energy very quickly. My mother was very diligent in keeping grown-up arguments and upsets away from me and my brother. She protected us from any upset by reassuring us that nothing was wrong and that everything was fine. The trouble was that it was not true and there were occasions when things were very much not OK. I am not saying that parents should download all their stuff onto their children, but learning ways to be honest about the emotional stuff that passes through is really important.

Parents and teachers assume that they are supposed to know all the answers and so when they don't have an answer they wing it. Don't you think it would be refreshing to explain to a child that 'Mummy or Daddy just had a bad or a sad feeling and, even though we don't know why, it's OK'? Not only does this honesty allow the child to trust their own feelings and intuition about a situation, it also teaches them that it's OK to have feelings that they don't understand, that they are still going to be OK, and that those feelings will pass.

Being protected from what my parents were feeling felt to me like being lied to. It was not necessary for me to know the details of what was going on, but I felt that something was wrong. When I knew something was wrong, being told that everything was OK and that it was all in my imagination went against my intuition and I began to doubt myself and later to feel unheard and not believed. To be told that everything was fine contributed to my feeling of not being understood.

The power of authority

It seems to me to be totally logical that if we spend the rest of our lives limited by the beliefs and decisions which we made when we were children, then teaching children how to process their emotions and release their traumas at an early age will result in far fewer problems for them later in life.

If dis-ease is the embodiment of unprocessed trauma, held in place by our perceptions and triggers, then learning to listen to your emotions and physical symptoms early on would set you up to prevent dis-ease rather than having to deal with the consequences later.

> *If dis-ease is the embodiment of unprocessed trauma, held in place by our perceptions and triggers, then learning to listen to your emotions and physical symptoms early on would set you up to prevent dis-ease rather than having to deal with the consequences later.*"

Children model what they see, not what they are told. They subconsciously observe and download information. If you try telling a child to be calm and respectful, yet display frustration and anger, it is the latter behaviour that will be stored for future reference. I remember being taught in my teacher-training courses that 'A noisy teacher makes a noisy classroom.' It is true that children need desirable behaviour modelled to them, by family and by their teachers and other grown-ups with whom they come into contact.

Schools and stress

If children model behaviour, picture the stressed schoolteacher. Children who are shown one thing and told another become very disillusioned with authority. The problem is, those in authority think they should have the answers, when really they are struggling with their own belief systems, stressors and triggers. The word 'stress' is a generic one, but we each have our own responses to pressure, deadlines, overwhelm and workloads. The more stress teachers are put under to meet performance targets, the more they feel overwhelmed and the harder it becomes to model the qualities that teachers are expected to instil in the children and students that they teach.

When I worked with a local school to introduce some simple stress-management skills, I began by running a series of 'Staff Stress Management' workshops, although the aim was to provide skills for the students. When we examined what core beliefs were running for the 14 staff who participated, it became clear that most of the staff were battling to hold themselves together during times of pressure.

If the people who are setting the example are struggling to manage their own thoughts and emotions, and their thresholds and health are compromised, is it any wonder that this results in a generation that becomes disengaged and disillusioned, becoming further withdrawn and uncommunicative? Disengagement is a classic coping mechanism in the face of stress.

Knowing how to process thoughts and feelings in the moment so that equilibrium is quickly restored is one aspect of emotional self-management. This, combined with working on your limiting beliefs and the structure of your belief system and on how you make sense of the world, is the counterpart to health and wellbeing. This extends even further into how we react and interact socially and globally.

Spread it about

Have you ever been smiled at by a radiant and charismatic person - a real smile, with sparkling eyes and a warm glow? Sitting in the space of someone who feels happy and content can have a calming and relaxing effect, just as sitting in the space of someone who is anxious or angry can also have a negative impact.

The Institute of HeartMath[48] has undertaken research into heart energy and heart coherence, and has measured the heart's electro-magnetic field, which may extend outside of body by over three metres (ten feet). Imagine then, that whenever you are within three metres (ten feet) of another person's heart, you are in their energy field and, of course, they are in yours. We always knew this intuitively; now it has been demonstrated scientifically.

Although this book is aimed at giving you the power to change your own health, there is a much bigger picture to consider. We have examined how traumatic events and the subsequent thoughts and triggers can impact on

---

48 See *www.heartmath.org/research*

your own health and life, but your health is influenced by others and you have an effect on other people. This is the ripple effect that we mentioned earlier (see *Family dynamics*, p. 203).

We have talked mostly about the body-mind connection or about how our perception interprets the world around us. This in turn sends messages to the body to react and to adapt, in order to compensate for the pressures and demands that are made upon us. These demands are personal and, if they are not managed or processed, they can become embodied and have an impact on our health and quality of life.

There are many components to a healthy life. In order to maintain health we must balance work, life and social commitments and ensure that there is time to allow the body and mind to rest and repair.

From the moment you are born, you are thrust into a world in which you must adapt and survive - from birth and learning in the first few years with family and primary carers, to school and your first social situations. We learn quickly how to behave and to respond with our peers and people in authority and we take this knowledge with us into our adult life.

Taking responsibility is the first step to being able to bring balance into the areas that you can affect. Changing what you can change and accepting what you can't change can help you to improve your health and life. This in turn can help change the circumstances of those around you, and the ripple effect flows outwards.

To be fully healthy, you need to be able to assess when you are not healthy and when you are unhappy. So becoming the observer of your own life is crucial, if you are to decipher what is and what is not working. Starting with the subtle, and sometimes not so subtle, messages from your body is the direct route to being able to pinpoint your specific thoughts and beliefs. When should you start to do that? Well, there is no time like the present!

10. It's never too late

"The great secret that all old people share is that you really haven't changed in seventy or eighty years. Your body changes, but you don't change at all. And that, of course, causes great confusion."

Doris Lessing[49]

There is a lot of information in this book, so you would be forgiven if you have got to this point and wondered how all this actually applies to you. After all, this is the kind of thing that 'other people' do - not 'ordinary people' like you, right? Well, that is how I used to feel, and I can tell you from experience that the message in this book applies to everyone – including you. You don't have to create a whirlwind to make changes that will benefit your health and bring more peace and happiness into your life. Small steps in the right direction will change your trajectory. The first step to making a change is to know that there is a choice.

Your body is an expression of what you think. No matter what your age, your body has the blueprint to be healthy. The trouble is that the older you get, the more you accumulate experiences that support your negative beliefs and the more this is expressed in your body.

I hope you might start to realise just how extraordinary you are and how intelligent and supportive your body is. All the aches and pains, all the illness and dis-ease is a response to getting you through life situations that you have found difficult. I urge you not to add insult to injury by condemning your amazing body for the way in which it has been responding to your thoughts and perceptions. Given the right conditions, your body can express your health and happiness, rather than your doubts and fears.

---

49 Writing in *The Sunday Times,* London (10 May 1992)

Inherited dis-ease, inherited beliefs

It is time to update your outdated belief system and, even if you don't have the inclination to research into the newest and latest findings in biology and science, at least be open to the concept that you are not a victim of your genes and past family patterns.

It is true that there may be a lot of energy in a belief. It may be so deeply rooted that you cannot imagine what life could be like without it, but that does not mean that your limiting belief cannot be changed.

> " *You may have an illness that you have had all your life or ever since you can remember. Should this mean that it is too late to change things now? No, of course not. It has only been the belief that your illness is inevitable, inherited or irreversible that has held it in place* "

You may have an illness that you have had all your life or ever since you can remember. Should this mean that it is too late to change things now? No, of course not. It has only been the belief that your illness is inevitable, inherited or irreversible that has held it in place.

It is true that over time the amount of energy that you have put into your illness may mean that the amount of repair your body now has to undergo in order to return to full health can be equally intense. If you have worn your body out with massive amounts of stress, toxins or ongoing physical trauma, you may feel that you will need to go through a lengthy programme of healing and repair to make things better. However, does this mean that you should not start to make those necessary changes right now and give your body the chance to get on with the healing process?

Now that you know dis-ease is a process, what can you do to guide and nurture it through the process, in order to return to health? What can you do to prevent re-triggering the process again? These changes can be made at *any* age and at *any* stage. It is never too late.

206

Hold that thought

What kind of thoughts would you like to hold? If the thoughts you would consciously like to hold are battling with your actual, subconscious thoughts and beliefs, maybe it's time to make some changes. The bigger changes may seem out of reach at the moment, but that doesn't mean you can't make little changes, create new habits and gain new and more resourceful perspectives in your life.

META-Health principles allow you to step off the treadmill of never-ending repetition and become aware of where you are in the dis-ease process. Then you can assess what you need to do to complete it. You have control.

What would you like to change? Although I would suggest that you are realistic in your immediate expectations, it doesn't mean that you cannot have a long-term goal and create a plan to move towards full health, even from the most complex of illnesses. Focusing on a positive future projection brings a powerful energy to your actions. I don't mean only positive affirmations and daydreaming. I mean that, if you truly believe that an outcome is possible, you will equip yourself to explore the means to get you there. The avenues to change are not shut down. You will notice that, once you begin to believe that things are possible for you, you will see more evidence to support that view. There is a part of the brain that is responsible for separating out things that are relevant to you from things that are not – it is called the 'reticular formation'. The function that modulates delivery of information to that part of the brain is called the 'reticular-activating system' or RAS. It works by changing how you notice new things when something becomes relevant to you. For example, you buy a yellow car and, suddenly, everyone seems to be driving yellow cars! You didn't notice them before, but now they seem to be everywhere. They were always there before, of course, but because they were not relevant to you before, your RAS simply filtered them out.

Resources that might help you to heal and return to a healthy life can, for some people, fall into the category of 'not relevant to me' and therefore are filtered out. It's not that such things are seen and dismissed, they are literally not experienced at all – they do not exist to the person to whom they

207

have no relevance. Once you awaken to a wider perspective, a new world of possibilities will open up to you.

You may think that you are 'just getting old', that it's too late or that your illness is too far advanced for you really to make a big difference to your health. Perhaps you might look at the category you have assigned yourself to and choose a different category instead, one that offers you better prospects, more resources and more health and happiness.

There are many contributing factors to bodily aging, just as there are many factors that affect someone's general threshold of health. But by far the biggest factor contributing to aging is what goes on in your mind. I don't suggest that you try to turn back the clock or expect to re-live your teenage years. However, I do suggest you start to accept where you are in your life and your health and to love and appreciate your body for looking after you so far. Then you will be able to accept that it's time to give your body a break for bearing the burden of your beliefs up until now. Accept each ache and pain as an indication that at some point you didn't feel strong enough or good enough; accept each illness as the manifestation of your emotional struggle and perhaps take some steps to release the weight of those stones that are weighing you down. You will be very surprised how much lighter, freer and, yes, younger you will feel, if you do.

Inside every unhealthy person

You could say that inside every unhealthy person is a healthy person trying to get out. No matter whether the illness is physical or psychological, within that illness is a person who is struggling with the symptoms and the emotion and energy of the original trauma that began the dis-ease process. With each incident in life where you have felt helpless and have feared a threat to your survival - whether it was a literal or a perceived one - a stone is added to the cumulative burden of those traumatic events that weigh you down and are affecting your buoyancy and health.

Some people do not wish to revisit past events; they would much prefer to forget them. However, the more you avoid something painful from your past and the more you try to forget it without accepting it, the more your subconscious thoughts and beliefs will try to adjust your body to compensate. If the events of which you have a conscious memory and the events that trauma has committed to amnesia remain in your system, your vital life force will be affected.

Be sure to like what's in your closet

If you want to be truly healthy, it's time to accept your past. The past is no longer happening and, in any case, your past need not predict your future. You may have hung onto the belief that you cannot change things from the past, so you just have to live with them. Well, that's half-true, of course. You cannot change things in the past, but for that very reason it makes no sense to go on living with them. It's time to let them go! I appreciate this is easier said than done, but there are techniques that will assist you in this process. You can release the traumas and triggers that keep you trapped in a dis-ease process. If there are any skeletons or demons in your closet, making friends with them, and accepting them for the past learning events they are, will be transformative for you and for your health.

If you want to transform your body from a prison to a temple, I cannot emphasise too often that the first step is to respect and be grateful to it. You cannot easily heal something you hate or feel betrayed by. Such emotions carry vibrations that will lay you low in depression and illness. With every small thing you release and change, you will shift your vibration to a higher level and feel increasingly lighter.

Try this simple exercise when you are feeling low, tune into what upsets you, look up and smile. Don't worry about changing your emotions, just change your face and smile, just as you would give a full-face smile when you are happy. The body does not know the difference between a fake and a real smile and you will release the same chemicals as you would when you are happy. Did you notice how your thoughts changed when you smiled?

When you are low and in the midst of pain and suffering, it is difficult to remember that there is another perspective and that there is always a choice. Sometimes a simple exercise like this one can shift your energy enough to remind you that you are more resourceful than you might previously have thought.

Pain may be necessary, but suffering is a choice

I would never wish to belittle anyone's pain, but pain is relative. It is something we all experience at some time and to some degree, but for some it is a way of life. I have great respect for those who must endure great amounts of pain in life, whether it is constant and chronic pain or acute pain. Such pain can be totally debilitating. However, have you noticed that not all people who have great pain consider themselves a sufferer? Not all people who have to live with pain as a constant in their lives become depressed, low or weighed down by their debilitation. Why would that be? Look at people like David Pelzer, one of the first people to write about his abusive childhood in his book, *A Child Called 'It'*[50]. David now enjoys a happy and loving family life and is a highly successful life coach. Or Simon Weston OBE, the Falklands War veteran who survived 49 per cent burns and 12 per cent wounds to his body and has endured over 70 reconstruction operations. Simon now lives a happy, fulfilling and inspiring life, working in the media and for charity. Despite the traumas both of these men have endured, their state of health is determined by their current, positive outlooks.

> *You have a choice only if you know what are the other options available to you.*

This brings us back to belief systems and the need to be specific about why someone has a pain or why someone has depression. It brings us back to how a person has handled past events in their life and how they have processed, released or held onto their traumas. If you are depressed, there is a reason for that. All the different aspects of your life - your diet and exercise, your environment, your behaviour and your thinking - will contribute to how healthy you are right now. So, the challenge is to think about what you can change sooner rather than later. You can start by making a list of what you could change more easily – right now? - and what needs more work.

---

50 *A Child Called "It" - One Child's Courage to Survive*, Dave Pelzer, Health Communications Inc., New York, 1995

The epidemic of fear

If you live in fear, you will find it very difficult to be resourceful. Fear is an exhausting state to be in. It is not possible to function properly in a 'fight or flight' mode. The thinking part of the brain is shut down in favour of the resources needed to escape or to fight. So, in fear, you cannot be creative.

You have a choice only if you know what are the other options available to you. So now that you understand that you and your body are operating as one and are, in fact, aspects of the same thing, perhaps you can start to act on behalf of your body and as if it were a valuable asset instead of a nuisance.

You can't run from yourself, no matter what you want to change. To allow change you have to truly accept things the way they are. If you are in any form of denial of, or resistance to, the truth of how things are or have been, it becomes very difficult to let them go and to move on. Fear prevents this kind of total acceptance, this bigger-picture perspective that takes you out of a 'small' position and into an enlightened position.

Fear brings helplessness and a victim mentality, but to release that fear you need to delve beneath the surface and find out what you are really afraid of. What is driving you and triggering your behaviour? Some people can do this on their own, others need professional guidance in the process.

So you can't see the wood for the trees?

If you feel that life is too overwhelming at the moment and you don't know where to start, adopting the META position can give you a new perspective and some breathing space, in order to disassemble the complex picture of your limiting beliefs into more manageable parts. It might help to begin by looking at different areas of your life such as:

- Home and family
- Relationships
- Work and career
- Friendships.

If you have multiple symptoms that are causing you distress, or if you don't quite know what is wrong but simply know that you are unhappy, keep a detailed daily diary of your emotions for a month. An analysis of the ebb and flow of your emotions, as revealed in your diary, will help you to spot the patterns.

The trick is to tackle your triggers one at a time. You are aiming to become fully aware of your own behaviours and responses, so that you can recognise the signs in your own body and emotions. Your body and emotions are your guidance mechanisms and will flag up when something is wrong and needs addressing. It's not good or helpful to deny or to ignore the symptoms or your emotional responses. As we can see from the two phases of dis-ease, that can lead to becoming stuck in a process and create degenerative dis-ease.

You are the expert on you

Nobody knows your problems like you and you alone can heal yourself. This is a much overlooked and yet vital concept of healing. Whatever medications you take and whatever help you employ, in the end it is you who will do the healing. Just trust and listen to your body, your emotions and your intuition.

META-Health provides a big-picture framework, so that you can be fully resourced in all that you might need to know to return to health. It accommodates all healing modalities and techniques, and empowers you to take control of what needs to happen in order to restore your body to health. Understand that you are the person in charge; you are the one who is responsible for your own health and healing is the first big shift in consciousness that most people have to make.

Owning responsibility for your own health may be daunting and may take a little time for you to consolidate. Most people are not used to the idea that they can influence their health in such a direct way. We are taught to go to the doctor when we are ill and that she/he will fix us. But we mostly believe that the fixing process has nothing to do with us: the doctor, the medication or the intervention is expected to do the job. Everything is done to us, rather than with us or through us.

What about my doctor?

This is not to say that you should not have a good relationship with your doctor. On the contrary, it is very important. But it's not the doctor who heals you - it's you. It is far better for the doctor too if you are the one to take responsibility for your own healing. This allows him or her to use their expertise in an advisory capacity and actually to work with you, so that you can find your way through the dis-ease process and back to health. You are the expert on you and, if you pay attention to what is going on, you can fully engage with the doctor's expertise and achieve empowering results. More doctors than you realise would rather work like this. Very few doctors would prefer to throw pills or cream at you and bundle you out of the door if the health-care system gave them the choice.

So, take responsibility and work with your doctor. Doctors have a limited amount of time with their patients, so the more specific you are about your symptoms, thoughts and behaviours, the more accurate your diagnosis and treatment will be.

In future, I predict that we will be seeing an increase in the number of doctors who are trained in META-Health; they will be able to help their patients understand the two phases of dis-ease and to release the fear of degenerative illness and the life-sentence mentality that often accompanies certain diseases. In an ideal world, doctors will begin to use the META model to identify whether a patient is in the stress or regeneration phase of illness. Then, their treatment and advice would assist the process by giving the patient a clear picture of where they are in the process and what needs to occur for them to return to health. While working with the doctor to manage the symptoms, the patient who receives advice and support that enables them to work on the original traumas, thoughts and triggers that hold the dis-ease in place has a great advantage in their quest for a return to full health.

Choose life

Would you like to work in this way with your health-care professionals? Would you like to be given full support to empower you to integrate the advantages

> ❝❝ *I suggest you take a good look at what your body is really doing for you and make friends with it.*"

of modern medicine with the self-help and personal-development tools that have been proven to transform people's psychological and physical issues?

It's time to take stock and to see what you can do for yourself. The more you do for yourself, the more empowered you will feel and the more evidence you will give to yourself and to others that you are in control.

Let's face it: if you are struggling with an illness, at least some of what you have been doing has not been working. And, if what you have been doing isn't working, do something different! What do you have to lose in adopting the META-Health model in addition to your existing treatments? If your current model of health is working for you, far be it from me to suggest you change your view. But if it's not, here is a gift of light in the darkness of pain and dis-ease. I suggest you take a good look at what your body is really doing for you and make friends with it. If you can listen to your body, understand it and appreciate it, you will transform your health and your life.

Create a picture with options and possibilities

If you no longer see yourself as the victim, but instead realise that you can have an impact on your own health, more options and possibilities open up for you. All this, without losing what you already have. In fact, all the options you had before could potentially be more useful, now that you know how they fit into the overall picture. You can make plans and devise strategies for your health. You can take small steps and have big goals. You can work with what you have going on right now, while at the same time going back to the events and traumas that need releasing and resolve those issues forever. From a META position, it is possible to prioritise; you can change the things that you are able to change and come to terms with the things that you can't. With a plan, you can organise yourself to maximise your healing potential.

There are very powerful tools that you can use to make these changes. I can say, from personal experience, that having them to hand and just knowing that they are available is a big step to emotional self-management and control and opens the gateway to robust and resilient health. Working with powerful tools for change is uplifting, enlightening and empowering, and I strongly believe that such techniques should not only be taught in schools, but offered through all medical practices. Once taught, they are skills that each person can own for themselves – with them, you are truly resourced and in control of your own mental, emotional and physical health.

11. When the pain of staying the same...

"The human animal is designed to experience, endure, survive and learn from traumatic episodes. If we did not possess this ability the human species would have become extinct."

David Berceli[51]

META-Health is not a healing modality or a technique in itself. It is a root-cause analysis tool that makes the connection between current symptoms and their original, root causes. However, the point at which you understand what your body is doing, why it is doing it and where you are in a process of dis-ease, is often when healing can start.

Making the change from victim to creator of your own health is the first step to taking real control over your life. I will never forget the turning point in my life when I found META-Health and Emotional Freedom Techniques (EFT). The day I made that call to Karl Dawson really was the first day of the rest of my life - the first step to getting my life and my emotional, mental and physical health back.

It did not happen overnight, of course, and there have been some painful and frustrating stages along the way. However, with each breakthrough there is a new freedom and a new level of understanding and spiritual growth. The more I listen to my body and my emotions, the better my relationship with myself and the healthier and happier my life becomes. It is something I feel compelled to share.

---

51 David Berceli PhD, Founder of TRE (Tension and Trauma Release); see http://www.bodymindheartandsoulharmony.com.au/tension-and-trauma-release/founder-dr-david-berceli/

Be the change

Before discovering these techniques, I had struggled in frustration to change things in my life, to no avail. I was defensive of my position, angry about being misunderstood, about being taken advantage of and about being mistreated. I felt that the things that people were doing to me were unfair and that I was a totally helpless victim. My happiness seemed to depend on them stopping doing these things - changing the way that they behaved – and on things outside myself, but the more I fought to change those external things, the more disconnected I became from myself. This desperation led to alcohol abuse and a nervous breakdown. I was 'not myself', I did not like myself and I could not control myself. From inside the mess that I was creating, it was difficult to see any way forwards.

The centre of a whirlwind is called the vortex. It is the place in the very centre that is still and calm, but around which the whirlwind swirls. I would compare the point I was at to entering that vortex. It is the place of nothingness to which depression can take you, disconnected and aloof from the whirlwind of the emotions. It's the make-or-break place, where you are suddenly nothing and nothing means anything. And, from this place, you can realise that you are everything.

I was physically, mentally and emotionally unwell. I was using drink and drugs to escape; I was violent and uncontrollable; and although I did not want to die, I did not want to live either. The whirlwind that was my life had gone far beyond my control and I was the Tasmanian Devil creating the mess. What changed it? The realisation that it was all down to me. I did this; I made this ... and I can change this. I entered into the vortex - the stillness that was inside the fear and the pain. In that moment, I knew I needed help and that's when I looked online, searching for 'anger management', and found that there were all kinds of techniques available to give me that help.

Adopt the META position

When you are triggered into a feeling or behaviour, it is difficult at first to rise above the situation and to choose a different course of action. Despite all my practice, I still sometimes find it difficult, but then, we are all a work in progress. Even so, it is very helpful to at least know that there is a META position. There is a way to make sense of what is going on, a way in which the answers can be found and the problem can eventually be resolved. It is the same with symptoms and dis-ease.

> *Even though you may find yourself in the midst of the dis-ease process, knowing that there is a way to make sense of it all takes you out of the role of victim and gives you back the reins of control."*

Even though you may find yourself in the midst of the dis-ease process, knowing that there is a way to make sense of it all takes you out of the role of victim and gives you back the reins of control. Knowing the reasons behind your illness gives you the power to influence the process. It may take some practice, and you might not know everything you need to know in order to decipher your dis-ease, but you *do* have a framework and you *do* have resources to find out how to make changes. META-Health gives you the broader perspective and the clarity of the bigger picture. I offer you the ladder to the META view.

If, for even a short breathing space, you can step outside your pain, your despair, your difficult situation and see that there is more going on, you can find new options. If you can understand the reason behind what is going on, you become empowered with the tools to investigate the missing pieces of the puzzle. By rising above the puzzle, it becomes clear which piece is missing and, most importantly, it becomes possible to see all the pieces together, forming the whole picture.

You may already have some pieces of the puzzle but, until you step outside your problem, you might not even know what you don't know. It's not possible to solve your problem from inside it; a new perspective is required.

Which pieces are missing?

It is time to start putting together what we have explored in this book. Although this book is not a directory of dis-eases, nor a full, step-by-step, self-diagnosis guide, I hope that there is enough information to open you up to the idea that you can do more than you may have ever realised, to heal yourself and to affect your own health and wellbeing.

There are four pillars to success in taking responsibility for your own health and wellbeing:

> - **Pillar 1** The ten META-Health principles that provide the full perspective of health and healing.
> - **Pillar 2** The META-Health analysis, to identify your events and triggers and any contributing threshold factors.
> - **Pillar 3** The META-Health plan, to define the holistic action plan for positive change across all areas of your life.
> - **Pillar 4** Powerful change techniques that work at the subconscious and energetic level for deep and lasting change.

Pillar 1: Ten META-Health principles

Let us look at the ten META-Health principles again, now that we have explored each of them in more detail. These principles free you from the victim's position, of 'being done to', and elevate you to the META position, in which it is possible to begin to investigate what is *really* going on in your body, mind and state of social health.

1. There is an *order* and a structure to the development and evolution of the brain and organ tissues.
2. There is an order and a *structure* to the communication between the organ-brain-psyche.
3. The starting point of dis-ease is a *traumatic* life experience.
4. Dis-ease is a *process*, which takes place in two distinct phases.

5. Fungi, mycobacteria, bacteria and viruses are bio-logical *helpers*.
6. Every symptom has a bio-logical and psychological *meaning*.
7. *Awareness* of this connection is a prerequisite for personal growth and health.
8. There is a body-mind-spirit and social *connection*.
9. The individual is *responsible* for acquiring knowledge and for making her/his own decisions in regard to her/his own wellbeing.
10. *Self-healing* is integral to all therapies and treatments.

Pillar 2: META-Health analysis

Based on an understanding of the META-Health principles, the META-Health analysis explores the purpose of the presenting physical and psychological symptoms. By doing this, we can identify the reason for the bio-logical change and locate the original traumatic event at its root cause, together with the derived belief systems that are holding the dis-ease in place.

By exploring specific information, it is possible to ask very targeted and direct questions about the nature of the original event, allowing you to make the connections for yourself on a deep, subconscious level.

Let us explore the questions again with another example:

- **The complaint** - What is your complaint and symptoms?

  Preferably based on a doctor's diagnosis, what is the specific dis-ease and symptoms?

  Mia has had a chesty cough for two weeks.

- **Location** - What is the position and purpose of the organ tissue? What does it do?

What organ and tissue is affected and what is its purpose? By understanding what the tissue's purpose, it is possible to understand what job it is doing and why it has changed.

Mia's bronchi are inflamed with a viral infection.

- **Dominance** - Which is your dominant side?

Using a simple clap test to see which hand is uppermost and therefore dominant, it is possible to determine the person's laterality. The dominant side represents the equal partner, or people of equal status, such as siblings, colleagues, friends. The non-dominant side represents someone in a nurture position, either nurturing or being nurtured.

Mia is right-hand-dominant. Both sides of her chest are inflamed. The doctor said the right side was more congested.

- **Organ tissue** - What is the specific organ tissue and its associated brain layer?

Bronchial mucous membranes (mucosa) derive from ectoderm and are associated with the cerebral cortex brain layer.

- **Theme and conflict** - What is the theme of the brain layer and the specific organ tissue conflict?

Theme of the cerebal cortex is 'social, territorial and contact' and the conflict theme of the bronchial mucosa is territory fear – a fear that someone may come into your territory or space beyond your control, or a fear that someone may leave your territory or space beyond your control.

222

- **Adaptation** - What change does this tissue make in the stress phase (cell increase or cell decrease)?

The bronchial mucosa thins in the stress phase, thus thinning the walls of the bronchi and dilating the bronchial tubes to allow more air in quickly to confront or face up to the situation. The lining is repaired in the second phase once the danger has passed, when the lining swells and the viruses are engaged to assist in the repair process. This activity restricts the diameter of the bronchial tubes during the repair.

- **Timing and phases** - When did the symptoms start? Is there a time when they are worse, or better? Has there been a break in the symptoms? Where in the two phases are you? (Confirm which phase by other symptoms: hot or cold, active or sleepy, obsessive or supine?)

Mia's symptoms started two weeks ago with a wheezy, tight chest. Coughing started one week ago, with a break from coughing for about two hours yesterday afternoon.

We know that the symptoms of a chest infection are the activity of repair and the engagement of viruses, which occurs in the second, regeneration phase. Also, in the last two weeks, Mia has been hot and feverish, with a slight temperature and an occasional headache. She has been quite sleepy, preferring to stay in bed - these are all symptoms of the regeneration phase.

The two-hour break in Mia's symptoms yesterday could be the healing peak. This would give us a timing of just over halfway through the second phase - just after the healing peak. This tells us that the whole of the second phase is approximately four weeks, which in turn makes the stress phase also four weeks long. Therefore, the original trigger may have occurred approximately six weeks ago.

223

- **Posing the question** - Formulate the question that will assist you in locating the traumatic event or thought that triggered this dis-ease process.

We could ask Mia about the turning point.

About two weeks ago, just before your symptoms started, what was it that you felt better about, with regard to a fear you had had about someone entering or leaving your space beyond your control?'

Or we could ask her about the traumatic event.

What happened about six weeks ago, when you were afraid that someone was either going to enter or to leave your space beyond your control?

Mia had had a heated argument with her partner, just over six weeks ago, in which her partner said he was unsure that he was ready to be a father. Mia feared he would leave her. Just two weeks ago, however, his behaviour towards her and their baby daughter changed and he became more loving and more relaxed. This was an indication to Mia that things were OK and that he had decided not to leave.

- **Status** - What is the status of the process? Is the status stuck in first phase, second phase, re-triggered or re-occurring?

This is the third chest infection that Mia has had since the baby was born. This would suggest an original event - in which Mia either believed someone would leave, someone threatened to leave or in fact did leave - has been re-triggered, either by the partner's behaviour or by Mia's own thoughts.

- **META message** - What is the belief or core belief?

  With a little more questioning, it was possible to establish that underlying Mia's fear of her partner leaving is a core belief that she is unlovable and will always end up alone. This is associated with an early event in which her father and mother separated and she felt that it was her fault.

Once we have such information, it is possible to formulate a plan to release the pattern of the specific illness, so that the body can complete the two phases of dis-ease and return to health. It also becomes possible to work on the core beliefs that hold this, and possibly other illnesses, in place.

Pillar 3: The META-Health plan

The META-Health plan is like a lifestyle plan and is usually created between a META-Health coach and an individual client, but of course you can also create your own plan. Now that you have more information and can adopt the META perspective, I encourage you to take a good look at each of the following areas in your life and to devise your own META-Health plan. The purpose of the plan is to facilitate you taking responsibility for the changes that you can make, to empower you to own those changes and to allow you to see a way forwards, with tangible and immediately achievable steps and long-term goals. It addresses all the aspects of your life, where there could be stress that is directly contributing to your health issue and to the depletion of your threshold for resilience and overall wellbeing. It offers a workable plan of changes you could make immediately and gives structure to more long-term lifestyle changes.

Following this list is an introduction to the main tools that I use and teach to resolve problems in each area. I have indicated where I apply specific techniques.

What's your META-Health plan?

Even if you do not have a dis-ease, you may still wish to improve your health, so take a look at the following areas. What changes would you plan to make immediately, and in the future, to improve your overall health and wellbeing?

225

1. **Emotional** - Now that you have examined your health issues in the light of the META-Health principles, and conducted a root-cause analysis, you will be more aware of the emotional relationship between your symptoms and past events in your life. You will have more awareness of your triggers and of the patterns of repeated re-occurrence of your triggers. You will be able to observe your behaviour and responses much more clearly and mindfully.

   What areas of your life bring you emotional stress? What strategies and tools can you use immediately in the moment to calm yourself? How can you release the emotion in a stressful situation?

   For coping 'in the moment', I would normally prescribe and teach stress-management tools such as HeartMath[52], EFT – Emotional Freedom Techniques[53] and EmoTrance[54]. These are quick-response techniques that can diffuse the trigger rapidly.

   What are the underlying emotional causes of the issue that affect you? Can you work with a specialist on these issues to resolve the trauma and release the triggers? What work can you do yourself on these issues?

   The most effective tool I have found for this kind of in-depth work is in Matrix Reimprinting[55]. I also use Colour Mirrors[56], especially when it is difficult to find a specifically relevant memory or event.

2. **Mental** - What tools can you use to perceive your situation differently? How can you keep track of your thoughts so that you can be aware of your patterns and habits? What new information can you research, to widen your scope and increase your awareness?

---

52 See www.heartmath.org
53 See *Emotional Freedom Techniques for Dummies*, Helena Fone, op. cit.
54 See www.emotrance.com
55 *Matrix Reimprinting Using EFT*, Karl Dawson & Sacha Allenby, op cit.
56 See *www.colourmirrors.com*

It is useful to have a few tools to hand to remind yourself that your thoughts are only thoughts and can be changed. Making a daily diary of your thoughts is a good method of capturing this information.

3. **Environmental** - Is there anything in your immediate environment at home or at work that you could change in order to relieve your stress and assist your healing? This could include getting rid of chemicals that exacerbate your condition, changing your physical environment to make work easier, getting help with some jobs. Assess the ergonomics of your seating and examine your daily routines to make improvements in things like bending, lifting and sitting. Can you bring in anything to assist your healing, such as things to improve the airflow or the lighting?

Can you change the dynamics of a stressful situation to avoid sitting near a person who causes you distress? What can you do to change your environment to make you feel safer and meet your needs better?

This environmental aspect is often overlooked and yet can be one of the simplest areas to address. By assessing your daily environment in the new light of your META-Health analysis, it is possible to see where many changes can be made to assist healing.

4. **Spiritual** - What is the higher message in your situation? What lessons have you not been learning that will enable you to release your dis-ease? What tools can assist you in taking more quality, personal reflection time and assist you in gaining a bigger-picture view of your problem?

I would usually prescribe HeartMath, meditation, breathing exercises and visualisation techniques, to assist in lowering your stress and increasing practice to move into a quiet, personal space. When these skills are practised on a regular basis, it becomes easier to use them, in order to shift your focus into a quiet space when under pressure.

5. **Physical** - Is there any exercise, such as stretching, qigong, yoga or walking, that you could do to assist your healing and mobility? Would massage ease your pain or improve your symptoms? What form of gentle exercise could you commit to do for just five or ten minutes a day that would begin to improve your mobility or flexibility?

    As a Chinese Health Qigong Instructor, I usually teach my clients some simple qigong exercises. This most often consists of some stretching exercises from the sequence *Ba Duan Jin*[57] and some standing and breathing qigong poses.

6. **Diet** - What changes can you make to your food and drink intake that will positively affect your healing? Which foods and supplements will create the best environment for optimum health? Do you need to drink more water?

    In most cases, I would usually recommend a high-alkaline, non-combining diet. You can find out more about the 'META-Diet' from META-Health coach Lene Hansson's website[58].

Working with your META-Health analysis

The META-Health plan would be discussed and designed with your META-Health analysis in mind. This means there would be a specific target of reducing symptoms and improving health over a period of time. Working with the two phases in this plan is very important - remember, the aim is not to relieve symptoms by simply suppressing them, but to assist you to complete the disease process and return to health.

There are many factors to take into consideration in managing a very serious illness. As some symptoms occur in the regeneration phase, it is necessary to plan with an individual how to manage the symptoms and to maintain a healthy threshold as they work through the two phases.

---

57 See *Ba Duan Jin: Eight-section Qigong Exercises*, The Chinese Health Qigong Association, Beijing, 2008, for a description of the basic movements.
58 *META-Diet*, Lene Hansson, Denmark, e-book, available from *www.lenehansson.com*

Using medications

A META-Health coach will not advise you on your medication and will encourage you to work closely with your doctor or health-care provider as you work through your META-Health plan. It is important that your dosages are checked with your doctor as progress is made, so that the correct amounts are prescribed as your body changes and returns to health. The META-Health plan takes into consideration the use of medication; Megan Smith is a META-Health coach who is also a clinical pharmacist and will advise on the use and side-effects of prescription medication through the UK Medicines Advisory Service.[59]

The aim is to create a plan that will give you the full META view of your situation and provide you with a strategy to change your health. This involves a short-term plan for making immediate changes and coping strategies, as well as a long-term plan with a structure for deep change work and lifestyle changes.

As with anything we wish to succeed in, it may help to be accountable. Sharing your positive action plan with supportive and encouraging people will in itself change your energy around your issue. By sharing your plan with someone, you will have more conviction and increase your resources. More things are possible!

If you want to heal your body and to enjoy health, wealth and happiness, you cannot do this by ignoring your 'bad stuff' - it needs to be released. The energy therapy techniques that I use do exactly that. While allowing the thoughts, feelings, memories and emotions to be there and to come to the surface, these techniques allow them to keep moving so that they are released. Different techniques work in different ways, but what they have in common is that they work on the human-energy system at a deeper level, to bring about deeper change in body and mind. Energy flows where attention goes.

---

59 Megan Smith, UK Medicines Advisory Service, www.ukmas.co.uk

Pillar 4: Powerful change techniques

Throughout this book, I have talked about making changes - changing beliefs, responses, releasing triggers, releasing trauma. All of this is possible with the use of powerful change techniques.

I am qualified as a practitioner, therapist and trainer in a number of healing modalities and use these for my own personal development and with clients. The following list is a summary of the techniques I have found most effective and so use most commonly.

EFT - Emotional Freedom Techniques

As with anything we wish to succeed in, it may help to be accountable. Sharing your positive action plan with supportive and encouraging people will in itself change your energy around your issue"

EFT[60] is a form of meridian tapping, derived from acupuncture and traditional Chinese medicine. It was developed by NLP Trainer, Gary Craig[61], and works in a similar way to acupuncture, except that there are no needles. Instead, you tap lightly with your fingers on the meridian points, to stimulate the increased flow of energy or *Qi*. This input of energy moves stuck and blocked energy and stimulates the correct flow throughout the whole system. The other significant difference from acupuncture is that to clear the blocked energy of a specific issue, you focus on that issue and bring to mind the thoughts, feelings and emotions that surround it. Doing this while tapping on the meridian points releases those emotions and allows an effective shift in psychological, emotional and physical distress.

You tap on a series of key points that are most often the ends or junctions of the body's meridian lines. These points have been documented as more active and conductive, making input more effective.

---

60 For more information, see AAMET and AMT websites at *www.aamet.org* and *www.TheAMT.com*
61 *The EFT Manual,* Gary Craig, op.cit.

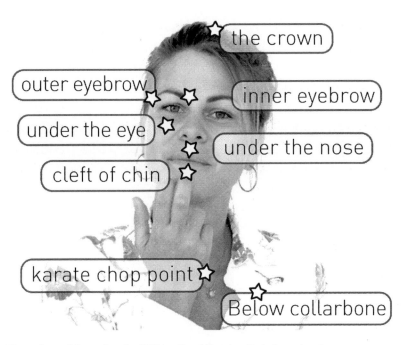

Fig.21 The main meridian points for EFT Emotional Freedom Techniques tapping

There is no correct sequence, although most commonly 'top to bottom' is used because it is easier. Imagine a simple, electrical circuit board. One of the components on the board, perhaps a bulb, is not working properly, because there is a fault in the circuit. The problem could be a faulty component somewhere else on the board, a short circuit, too much or not enough energy flowing properly. In order to get the bulb to work, the energy must flow properly through all components, so checking the flow of energy throughout the whole circuit is vital for correct and sustained energy flow.

This is how your body and mind work together. Your vital life force flows through your body on many levels. Great doctors and scholars over history have identified and mapped the patterns of electro-magnetic flow. This energy extends from the quantum level within every atom of every cell, to the cells and the tissues, the central nervous system, the meridian system and out to the chakra system. It is even possible to measure the electro-magnetic field, with special bio-field imaging technology.

Working with this energetic system brings very deep and lasting change, as it affects you on all levels. Tapping on the meridian points, while allowing the emotion to arise, allows the energy of the emotion to be released. This in turn allows the information trapped in the energy to be released. The release of this information often brings about great realisations for people and leads to a clear reframing of the original perspective. It is not about 'tapping out' or 'getting rid' of the problem - it is more significant than that. Tapping through an issue brings great acceptance and understanding of that issue, allowing for a more resourceful and balanced perspective.

Matrix Reimprinting using EFT

Matrix Reimprinting[62] was created by EFT Master Karl Dawson, when he realised that you could actually 'step into' a memory and tap on the earlier version of yourself in that memory. Karl has pieced together discoveries emerging from various new sciences, so that Matrix Reimprinting provides a clear picture of how the mind and body work together, how we store memories, and how we tune into those memories when triggered. This technique has a very powerful and profound effect. Unlike standard EFT, in which you must associate with and feel the emotions and the feelings of the original event, Matrix Reimprinting means that you can remain 'disassociated' and yet immediately release the trauma from your earlier self by imagining tapping on that self, back at the time of the original traumatic event. Since this technique was first introduced, there have been many developments - most notably the Matrix Birth Reimprinting protocol developed by Sharon King[63]. The Matrix Reimprinting technique continues to be one of the leading modalities in this field of personal development work. It is especially effective because it is possible to 'step in' and investigate earlier memories, and to ask your earlier self or 'ECHO' (Energy Conscious Hologram) what beliefs or decisions they made that day, as a result of what happened. You can also ask what other memories you need to go to, and what needs to happen to fully resolve the issue, and to create a positive learning experience from the event.

---

62 *www.matrixreimprinting.com*
63 *www.magicalnewbeginnings.com*

Matrix Reimprinting is especially effective in combination with META-Health, because you can work with a timeline of events, visiting each earlier version of yourself and resolving the trauma at its source. It still amazes me, when I work with someone on this technique, that we can resolve an issue that occurred many years ago and that the physical symptoms of the client beside me often change as we work. Proof indeed of the power of our amazing bodies!

EmoTrance – Emotional Transformation

EmoTrance[64] is an effective tool, like EFT in that it releases blocked energy back into the state of flow. It was developed through much experience and understanding of energy by leading energist, Silvia Hartmann. This technique achieves its results through the power of intention - by intending to 'soften and flow' the blocked energy. It works on the principle that everything is energy - all thoughts, emotions, feelings, pictures, memories; they are all information stored in energetic form to be tuned into and recalled, just as a computer recalls information from a database. It is when this information becomes stuck, is not updated or rewritten that we experience problems. This principle is true in general for EFT and for all energy work, but this technique really uses this principle to focus and to clear the issue.

Primarily, with EmoTrance you think about the problem and notice how it makes you feel in your body. You bring your awareness to that feeling and tell yourself, 'This is only energy.' In your awareness of this energy, you can intend it to soften and, as it softens, it can start to flow and move. As this stuck energy starts to move, you can invite it to exit the body wherever it needs to go, and continue to soften and flow the energy until it has all been released. You then focus again on the problem and see how it now feels. This 'soften and flow' technique is repeated until the energy of this issue has been released and you no longer get upset about it. Something quite profound happens with this technique, as with EFT. As the energy shifts, your thoughts, memories and understandings become clearer. As the energy is released, the information stored in that energy is freed for processing and there is a deeper understanding of the original problem. With this processing and learning,

---

64 *www.emotrance.com*

comes a positive gift and lesson from the issue, and it is possible to continue the process until an energised, positive end-state has been achieved.

HeartMath

HeartMath[65] is a coaching model, developed by the HeartMath Institute, which employs a range of techniques; the technique I use the most is heart-focused breathing.

This breathing technique works very quickly to bring about balance in the body and mind and, in particular, to synchronise the heart and the mind. It works by shifting the heart's activity from a disordered pattern into an ordered and coherent sine-wave. Once the heart is in the sine-wave, the mind and the rest of the body synchronise. There are three stages to shifting into 'heart coherence':

1. Place your hands on your heart and bring your attention to your heart.
2. Begin to breathe evenly in for five counts and out for five counts and imagine the breath going directly in and out of your heart.
3. Once you are settled into this breathing pattern, bring to mind something that makes you feel love, gratitude or appreciation.

By maintaining this breathing technique and focusing on a positive emotion, the strength of the sine-wave increases and not only has a greater effect on the body and mind, but can also synchronise the heart patterns of the people around you.

---

65 HeartMath Institute, *www.heartmath.org*

Colour Mirrors

Developed by intuitive healer Melissie Jolly, Colour Mirrors[66] is a more recent addition to my tool kit - and what a powerful and exciting addition it has been.

Colour is vibration and, as vibrational beings, we respond to colour on a very deep level. Although your body appears to you as being solid, it is in fact composed of particles vibrating at a frequency that makes it appear to be solid. This is a concept that is difficult to get your head around, I know. It is a scientific fact that bypasses most people. The Colour Mirrors system of coloured bottles and sprays works with your energy system to tune you into your stored information. By working with the colours or combinations of colours that you are attracted to or that make you feel uncomfortable, you can very quickly uncover and clear issues. As with other energy work, when you focus on an issue and clear the energy of it, the issue itself and the problems associated with it become clearer; it is then possible to take a new, uncluttered perspective in which you can be more balanced and resourceful.

Chinese Health Qigong[67]

The elegant stretching and relaxing movements of Health Qigong bring the body, mind and spirit into alignment. The practices that I teach have roots in Chinese history dating back over 2,500 years.

By focusing on a series of specific stretching techniques, the body can release blocked energy and the mind can be calmed. As the body and mind become synchronised, a connection is made that is experienced as a spiritual awareness – a feeling of being very present and in the moment. The physical aspects of these specifically designed movements have been analysed in sport-science research and are proven to bring greater movement, flexibility, strength and suppleness.

I often combine qigong with EFT, EmoTrance, HeartMath breathing and Colour Mirrors in my treatment, with amazing results.

---

66 *www.colourmirrors.com*
67 See *http://jsqg.sport.org.cn/en/* or *http://www.deyin-taiji.com/what-is-health-qigong*

TRE – Tension and Trauma Release exercises

TRE (Tension and Trauma Release)[68] -exercises are an amazing tool developed by David Berceli. They are a series of simple exercises that induce gentle fatigue in key muscle groups, thus engaging the body's natural mechanism for releasing the freeze response, just as animals do in the wild. Through the gentle fatigue, and then relaxation, of these muscle groups, you are able to take control over the body's built-in, self-regulating, trauma-release mechanism, allowing for a purely physical release of stress, tension and trauma. This is a powerful addition to my tool kit, since it does not require a conscious awareness of the original trauma events or triggers, but relies on the body's innate ability to self-regulate.

There can be many aspects to a problem, some immediate and acute and some long-term, that deplete your energy reserves and affect your health threshold. It is important to recognise these effects and to adopt the best way of balancing and replenishing your energy.

What are you not letting go of?

When I was at my lowest ebb, in fatigue and depression, I was living in fear and anger. Both were a result of feeling totally helpless and frustrated. I was afraid of losing what I had, hurt and angry at not being able to get what I wanted and afraid of not being in control. All these heavy, negative emotions were creating a cycle of behaviour that of course made everything worse. In a constant state of 'fight or flight' and panic, I was triggered into rage, hysteria or deep depression, and so my behaviour put me at great risk of realising my deepest fears. There was nowhere to run and nowhere to hide. I could not hide from myself. It was myself that I could not control. My view of the world had twisted and I couldn't see things clearly. I was fighting against everything, resisting what I thought other people were doing to me. All my attention was going into thinking and obsessing over all the things that other people were doing.

---

68 TRE (Tension and Trauma Release) exercises, see *http://traumaprevention.com/*

When it comes to working on emotional issues, some people will not be ready to let go of certain aspects - especially if the emotion is anger. The question to ask yourself is, 'Are the things that I am thinking or feeling good for my health, or detrimental to my health?' Because at the end of the day, no matter what anyone else has done to you or tries to do to you, your thoughts and your feelings are your own. *You* create them, *you* control them and *you* have the power to change them.

Whatever you decide to do to change or to resolve a situation, how you feel and think is your responsibility and it has the biggest impact on your health and your life, without exception. Your life situation might not be ideal; things may not be the way you want; people may be making your life difficult: but they do not create your thoughts and it is your thoughts that create your health.

If you want to make a change without, you have to go within. External stress that is imposed on your system can have an effect only if you allow it to. Shifting your position from victim to being empowered comes from a shift in perception first. If you can understand why you are unwell, why you feel and react the way you do, you are open to feeling more compassion and tolerance for others. This in turn lifts you out of the role of victim. It's not about you! The way someone treats you, or talks to you, is not about you. It's your own stuff that makes it about you and, if you can learn to do that to yourself less and less, things do change.

What makes you feel empowered?

Gaining control can be both exhilarating and daunting. Responsibility is not something that everyone is ready for. However, once you start to notice and recognise how your health issues are connected to your emotions and thoughts, it becomes increasingly difficult to ignore that connection. We have access to oceans of energy and a blueprint for health that the body can return to. Doing everything in your power to allow the proper flow and balance of energy and health is a lifestyle choice, and the stronger and more robust your system becomes, the greater the reward and the easier the changes become too.

A change on one level is a change on all levels. If you address your environment, it will impact your health in many ways. Just as if you change your perception of a situation, what was once a trigger can no longer send you into the biological-psychological-social turmoil that it once could. Small changes allow for bigger changes and you will notice a new relationship with yourself developing.

No time like the present

You are always more powerful with more resources, so I encourage you to find out more for yourself. By its very nature, self-development has to be experienced directly. Health must be experienced and each person must make his or her own connections between body and mind.

You have a choice to be pro-active and positive - or not. I make no judgments about anyone who finds the idea of becoming master of their own life and their own health a daunting prospect. For some, the idea of health is so far out of reach that the overwhelming sense of not knowing where to start is itself a trigger into an entire system of negative beliefs. Remember that you are not alone and there is a huge network of people out there taking steps, even if they are small, tentative ones, to actively engage in their physical, mental and spiritual healing.

The next remarkable stage of your journey has begun with this book. All that is required is the intention to make a change. With that intention, your sights are aligned to move you to where you want to be. It all starts with you and ends where you allow it.

Conclusion

"Anyone who stops learning is old, whether at twenty or eighty. Anyone who keeps learning stays young. The greatest thing in life is to keep your mind young." **Henry Ford I**[69]

S tress is a part of everyday life. It is a natural reaction of the body to respond to stress and to compensate for the changing demands that we encounter every day. In order to manage and meet those demands, we constantly go through subtle physical and psychological shifts, always seeking to return to balance and equilibrium. Our minds and bodies are remarkable creations and never cease their constant search for resolution to our problems. Sometimes our traumas and our anguish are caused by the world not living up to our expectations. At other times, they develop because the world does live up to the low expectations formed by our limiting beliefs from early childhood experiences. To go through these traumas and difficulties is to grow and to become stronger.

Personal growth

However, we can only grow from challenges if we can move through them. If you are experiencing dis-ease, it is most likely that you are trapped in a cycle of re-triggering your past, painful experiences and it is this that is causing your body to change. It is no longer assisting you in a temporary, subtle adaptation; it is now 'hanging' in the same way as a computer program 'hangs' in a repeating cycle, unable to complete its task and exit.

If you have been 'stuck in a rut', unable to change your situation because you felt a victim of circumstance or of your ill-health, I hope you have by now awakened to the possibility that all is not lost.

69 *My Life and Work - An Autobiography of Henry Ford*, Henry Ford, Classic House Books, New York, 2009

> *We can only grow from challenges if we can move through them. If you are experiencing dis-ease, it is most likely that you are trapped in a cycle of re-triggering your past, painful experiences and it is this that is causing your body to change.*

When I found META-Health, I was pretty much as lost as you can get. I was on the verge of giving up and was hopelessly looking for something - anything - to relieve my emotional and physical pain. I did not believe for one minute that my life could be turned around so fast. With a combination of META-Health, EFT and Matrix Reimprinting, I transformed my mental, physical and emotional health and ultimately my life. I now have the perfect relationship and my dream career. It is part of my life development always to remember what it was like in those dark times and how I got to that stage in my life. In part, this is in order to share with others the way to freedom, but also to remind me that the mental and physical illness I experienced holds the key to my deepest personal and spiritual development. My struggles have made me stronger. My dis-eases were the key to my way out, opening the door to a new life.

How did this work for me? I began with EFT, 'tapping' on everything, especially the anger, frustration, and fear. For each situation that was triggering me, I used EFT to release my energy, like letting out steam from a pressure cooker. Every emotion that overwhelmed me, I tapped and I tapped. Often I cried, I screamed and I shook - sometimes I even laughed. As I began to find a little more calm, I was able to come back into my body and to become aware of my symptoms - my bad back, my indigestion, my overweight, my acne, and, most importantly, my fatigue and my mood swings. For each symptom, I used the META-Health model to discover my triggers. This understanding brought about an enormous transformation in my view of myself - not only that, it gave me a plan to work with. I used EFT and Matrix Reimprinting to locate the original memory and, with these amazing techniques, I was able to release original trauma stuck in my system. In turn, this resolved the situation, allowing for a deep and clear understanding of what the original trauma had been and the beliefs and decisions that I had formed at the time of the trauma.

As I released these traumas and learned about the way I perceived the world, my dis-eases began to heal. This sometimes happened instantaneously with the release of the trauma; sometimes, it needed more work as I explored more complex aspects of my symptoms and behaviour. In learning about these tools and adopting this understanding, I have claimed back my life and transformed my health. This doesn't mean I never get sick at all, but it does mean that I now know why! I mentioned an example of this on the first page of this book when I talked about developing a headache while talking to my book coach.

I laughed as soon as the headache struck me, even though it was quite painful. These aches and pains can tell you so much that you were consciously unaware of if you listen to them. How did I know what the belief and message was? Let's take a look.

It was a tension headache, in the muscles around the scalp, and I know that the theme of the musculo-skeletal system is 'being strong or good enough to do something'. Around the head, this thought can be linked to the intellect. I also know that this pain occurs in the second phase (when the issue is resolved and the swelling and healing take place). The headache started immediately after Kevin, my book coach, finished explaining how he would coach me. So what was the turning point that flipped me into the second (healing) phase? It was not what *he* said, it was what *I* thought that brought on the headache. I realised for myself that 'I can do this!' I felt this feeling deep within me; I knew I could do it! No sooner had I felt this than the headache started up. So, the question is: had I previously had the belief that I couldn't do it? Had I been thinking that I wasn't clever enough? Did I have a fear that I was not organised enough? Well, the answer was 'Yes' to all of those things, although it was not apparent to me until that point.

What a gift to be able to understand myself, to work on myself and to overcome and let go of those limiting beliefs. This new relationship with my body has gifted me many insights and I truly appreciate those gifts.

What would it be worth to you to be healthy? What cost could you put on a healthy, active and fulfilling life? What would it mean to you to be able to transform your dis-ease into health? For me, taking those first steps, learning more and finding these valuable tools has been priceless.

A new position

If you picked up this book because you wanted an answer to your health problems, I hope I have opened a doorway for you to see beyond the limitations that frustrate you. For some of you, this book will be enough to galvanise you into action - even if that action is to simply be more aware of just how amazing you really are. If you have made friends with your body through reading this book, I will be pleased that you have begun a new and potentially life-changing relationship with your greatest gift.

Others may find the information in this book a little overwhelming. After all, the human body is elegantly designed, but not necessarily simple to understand. I have deliberately included some of the complex aspects and trust that you will take what you need from this book on a conscious level, and absorb more on a subconscious level. Perhaps you will begin to experience subtle changes in your life that you may, if you think about it, be able to relate to a shift in your perception after reading this book. Having experienced first-hand the power behind the principles in this book, it is an honour and a privilege to share this information with you.

There may be some who find this book frustrating, because it does not offer individual answers to each illness. It does, however, offer in broad brushstrokes a picture of META-Health. It was not my intention to list every illness known to man or to create a directory of case studies. My specific aim was to outline the incredibly ordered way in which our bodies, minds and spirits work together and, through sharing my own journey, hopefully inspire you to take new or renewed steps towards your *own* health.

There is a purpose for every change in the body that may eventually express as dis-ease. Whatever the organ, whatever the tissue, there is a purpose and a process at work - it's up to you to pay attention to the message and, with this new information, you can decipher what that message is telling you.
By giving a few examples from each of the brain layers and showing how the

body is working intelligently to support you, I hope to have introduced the concept that your own illness has a specific starting point. It has a specific purpose and it passes through a definable process. Once you are aware of this, change is possible.

Write your own story

Perhaps there are things in your past that cause you pain, and no matter how you try to move on, your health has never fully recovered. Whatever your personal story, it is *your* story. And if it's your story, isn't it time to write one that you can enjoy a little more? Life is stressful and it is far too easy to become overburdened by demands on your time, to the point where something has to give. Don't let it be your health.

This book might be enough for you to make changes that transform your health or you may feel more inclined to maintain your health improvements with like-minded people. It's always a good idea to surround yourself with positive, like-minded people, who can encourage you when you are confused or when the going gets a little tougher.

> *Whatever your personal story, it is your story. And if it's your story, isn't it time to write one that you can enjoy a little more?"*

You may need some advice or have a specific question that this book didn't answer. Perhaps the information in this book has raised new questions that had not occurred to you before. Remain curious! It's not too late to claim back your health and vitality. It's not too late to find happiness and enjoyment in every day.

Everything you need

I was initially worried about how I would end this book, and then I realised that it is not an ending, it is a beginning. This is, as they say, the first day of the rest of your life. I hope that you have new thoughts and feelings and even excitement about what the future holds for you. When I started to work on myself, I began to see instant changes and within months I felt very different. Some deeper changes took longer and of course some things are ongoing. I am

243

privileged to have this wonderful information at my fingertips and a bulging tool kit of self-help techniques, which I use and enjoy sharing with others.

I have a passion for the META-Health introductory training, because it gives everyone access to the concepts in this book. I am always excited to share this information with a new group and to facilitate new people on their journey of self-discovery. This book is a taster of what I share in more detail in the two-day training course and, for those who wish to pursue it further, the Master Practitioner training.

Working together with a group, exploring questions about specific illnesses, about the dis-ease process, about how to apply these principles and how to make changes to your life is a great way to create a new path to health. In just two days, you can grasp the basic principles of META-Health and have the confidence to apply life-changing concepts to your own life.

It is exciting when new people get together and become part of the growing META-Health community. There are many therapists, counsellors, health practitioners, chiropractors, doctors and 'ordinary', wonderful people like you, all sharing their skills and expertise and contributing to the growing body of research that supports META-Health.

I hope that you have been as excited by this information as I was when I first heard it. I was hungry for more and I wanted to find out at once how I could apply this understanding to my own health and wellbeing. There is so much you can do right now from your already new perspective. Your awareness and META knowledge already gives you the first step to higher ground. Your next steps don't need to be complicated. Simply starting a new relationship with your body will begin the process of change.

Where you go next is up to you. Wherever you do go, I hope you will remain curious and open to the possibility that you are far more powerful that you could have ever imagined.

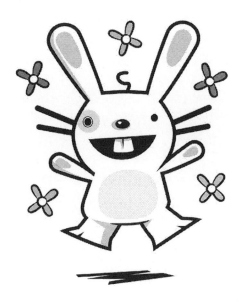

Fig.22 Happy Bunny

Praise for the two-day Introductory Training

'Having encountered Sam Thorpe on a few occasions prior to the introductory workshop on META-Health and knowing of her background as a teacher, I was convinced that she would be presenting this relatively complex and fascinating subject matter in a clear and concise as well as fun manner, and I was not disappointed!

A whirlwind of passion and energy, she also exudes compassion and enthusiasm for this relatively new discipline, is patient when answering any questions and clear in guiding us through the discussions and discoveries.

I found this workshop enormously beneficial on a personal as well as a professional basis. It gave me a hugely better understanding of why I have developed the dis-eases I have, but it goes far beyond that: in my opinion it is the hitherto (missing) link between the medical profession and energy psychology in that it gets to the source of where illnesses come from and why we develop them in the first place. The body-mind makes no mistakes...

In short, I urge anyone interested in energy psychology as well as complementary, alternative and traditional allopathic medicine or the social sciences to attend her course, even if they don't want to go on the full training as a META-Health coach. One thing is for certain: it's a new tool for me that I intend to use extensively in my professional life! After two days I left the training and my new-found friends (my fellow participants on the course) with my head buzzing from possible applications to clients and a deep respect for Sam Thorpe as a teacher and course leader.'

Anna Williamson, www.eftoxford.co.uk

'Sam's extensive knowledge, coupled with her infectious enthusiasm for this ground-breaking new model of health and wellbeing, make the course enjoyable and a great learning experience at the same time. As a result of this two day introductory course, I can really see the value of training as a health coach practitioner as it gives a therapist from any discipline detailed scientific and technical information that demonstrates the body-mind connection with medical evidence provided by brain scans. This provides the missing link between the intuitive way many therapists work and evidence-based medical treatment and makes a big contribution to the ongoing bridge-building between the gap of science and spirituality necessary for humanity to thrive rather than just survive in the 21st century. I recommend this course to anyone who wants to be part of this evolution.'

Amy Branton, www.freehearteft.co.uk

'As a result of this course my life will be different, because although I already know that my body is my friend, this course has really shown how that friendship works and it's amazing that a couple of days later I feel different about myself, especially about the anxiety and panic attacks that rear their heads every so often. I now really know what they are trying to show me and can go back to the cause with much more ease and root it/them out and work with them with EFT/Matrix.

I would recommend this course because of the fascinating content and the empowerment it will give you, it gave me. Plus, you will be in excellent hands with Sam, who is a trainer par excellence. Sam creates a great environment in which to learn that is warm and supportive. You won't think about your health in the same way when you have the information that this course gives you.'

Niall Morton, www.eft4u.co.uk

'Sam's Introduction to META-Health' workshop opened a new window of understanding on how we could use our physical symptoms to gain a greater understanding of our functioning as a whole being. It has enhanced my counselling practice as I am able to identify and ask informed questions relating to their circumstances, which has helped the client swiftly make sense of their world and to assist in making choices whether to and how to address their current situation.

Sam is extremely eloquent and knowledgeable and a very easy-to-understand teacher. Her pace respected the expertise that existed in the room (we were all counsellors) and we became animated as a collective as it clicked into place for us.

Thanks, Sam, for the opportunity.'

Claire Poole, www.therapysouth.co.uk

'I trained in META-Health with Sam and as a Psychotherapist found the training gave me invaluable insight and addition to my skill set. I am now able to help my clients identify triggers to a host of physical and psychological difficulties. This means that we are able to hone in on areas to explore and resolve in a much more efficient and accurate way. A must for all Counsellors and Psychotherapists.'

Sally-Ann Soulsby, BA (Hons) Psych, Dip. Couns., Dip. H. Couns., Dip. Psychotherapy and Hypnotherapy (UK), www.innerwisdom.co.uk

To find out more about META-Health and Introductory Training, and other training and services go to the website:
www.intoalignment.com

I look forward to meeting you on your journey to health.

Resources

If you would like to know more about some of the topics discussed in this book, here are some accessible titles to start you off on your journey of discovery – enjoy!

Dawson Church, Ph.D, *The Genie in Your Genes – Epigenetic Medicine and the New Biology of Intention, Energy Psychology Press*, Santa Rosa, CA, USA, 2008

Karl Dawson & Sacha Allenby, *Matrix Reimprinting Using EFT*, Hay House UK Ltd, London, 2010

Johannes R. Fisslinger, *META-Health, De-coding Your Body's Intelligence*, Fisslinger (Kindle e-book), 2013

Helena Fone, *Emotional Freedom Techniques for Dummies*, John Wiley & Sons Ltd, Chichester, 2008

Ryke Geerd Hamer. Med. Mag. Theol., *Scientific Chart of German New Medicine®*, Amici di Dirk, Ediciones de la Nueva Medicina S.L., Alhaurin el Grande, 2007

David R. Hamilton Ph,D, *It's the Thought that Counts – Why Mind over Matter Really Works*, Hay House UK Ltd, London, 2005

Silvia Hartmann, PhD, *Oceans of Energy – The Patterns & Techniques of EmoTrance*, Volume 1, DragonRising, Eastbourne, 2003

Bruce H. Lipton Ph.D, *The Biology of Belief – Unleashing the Power of Consciousness, Matter and Miracles*, Hay House Inc, Carlsbad, CA, 2008

Lynne McTaggart, *The Bond: Connecting Through the Space Between Us*, Free Press, New York, 2011

Lynne McTaggart, *The Field – The Quest for the Secret Force of the Universe*, HarperCollins, New York, 2002

Lynne McTaggart, *The Intention Experiment – Using Your Thoughts to Change Your Life and the World*, Free Press, New York, 2007

Patrick Obissier, *Biogenealogy – Decoding the Psychic Roots of Illness, Freedom from the Ancestral Roots of Disease* (English translation), Healing Arts Press, Rochester, Vermont, USA, 2006

Rob van Overbruggen, Ph.D, *Healing Psyche – The Patterns in Psychological Cancer Treatment*, Rob van Overbruggen, Ph.D, BookSurge Publishing, 2006

Dave Pelzer, *A Child Called "It" – One Child's Courage to Survive*, Health Communications Inc., New York, 1995

T.W. Sadler Ph.D, *Langman's Medical Embryology*, (11th ed.), Lippincott, Williams and Wilkins, Baltimore, USA, 2010

Robert C. Scaer MD, *The Body Bears the Burden – Trauma, Dissociation and Disease* (2nd ed.), Routledge, New York, 2007

Index

A

abandonment, 57, 58-59, 142

abdomen, 61

acne, 51, 145, 240

    facial, 41

acupuncture, 8, 230

adaptation(s), 53, 120, 137, 138, 139

    biological, **50-63**

    physical, 167

    psychological, 68

    short-lived, 139, 152

adrenal cortex, 36, 85

    underactive, 136

adrenal gland, 62

affirmations, 180

aggression, 101, 113, 10, 143, **148-50**, **157-160**, 163

    depressive, 162

    inward, 162

aging, 208

alcohol abuse, 7, 218

allergen, 124-5

allergy(ies), 48

    to coffee, 48-49

    to bright light, 118, 124, 130

    to foods, 124, 130

    to medications, 124, 130

    to noise, 118, 124, 130

    to peanuts, 170

    to smells, 118, 124

    to temperature, 118, 124, 130

alpha and beta islet cells, 86, 157

amnesia, 110, 209

anger, 50-51, **148-150**, 190, 194, 201, 236, 237

    conflict, 155-156

    indigestible, 130, **141-144**

    territory, **148-150**

    threat, 156-160

animal(s),

    social, humans as, 26, **42**

ankles, 142

annoyance, 176-178

anorexia, 149, 157-160, 162

anxious, 118, 128, 132, 133, 140, 149-150

appetite loss, 66

arms, 121

    pain in lymph glands of, 129

arteries, 36

    coronary, 36, 86

    narrowing, 119

arthritis, 89

association, 124

    technique, 93-94

asthma, 63, 70, 170, 199

authority, 51

    figure, 51

    power of, 200-201

autonomous nervous system (ANS), 62, 169

awareness, 167, 221

    of triggers, 226

    to increase, 226

axons, 126

Ayurvedic medicine, 44

B

back, 101, 121

    ache, 13, 104

bacteria, 31, 73,76, 79, 80, 81, 83, 90, 128, 220

Bader, Dr. Anton, xi, 29

balance, 9, 66, 152-154, 160, 187, 189

    in body and mind, 234

    restoring, 67, 68

    return to, 80, 120

behaviour(s), 157, 190, 212

    changing, 139, 140

    patterns, 197

    recorded, 171

belief(s), 58, 86, 104, 105, 107, **108-112**, 134-135, 166, 168, 179, 189-190

    'I am unlucky', 174

    being aware of, 101

    as baby, 121

    'cannot control my space', 132

    'cannot define myself/position', 132, 146

    'cannot escape', 132

    core, 99, 112, 186, 191-192

    'defiled', 144-146

    'deformed', 144-146

    'I don't understand', 135

    filters, 173

    forming, 178

    inherited, 117, 195,160, **206**

    learned, 169

    limiting, 200-201

    'must be perfect', 135

    'not fast enough/never will be

G

health, 32, 187

   blueprint for, 237

   compromised by tension, 184

   foods for, 228

   holistic, 22

   integrated approach, 30

   model of, 19

   normal, 72

   optimum, 228

   plan, 207

   professional, 11

   return to, 55, 58, 73, 80, 82, 135, 198 206

   state of, 65

   strategy to change, 229

   threshold, 17, 18, 82, 208

   transformed, 241

heart, 68

   attack, 90

   coherence, 202, 234

   energy, 202

   electro-magnetic field of, 202, 231

   rate, 65

HeartMath, 226, 227, 234

   Institute of, 202

heel pain, 96

helpers, biological, 31, 80, 221

helplessness, 62, 129, 132-133

hives, 124

hormones, 62, 154-162

hyperactivity, 66, 137

hypermobility, 121

hypnotherapy, 168

hypocondriac, 17

hypoglycaemia, 152

hypothalamic-pituitary-adrenal axis (HPA axis), 63

hysteria, 236

I

Illness(es), 13, 23,14, 17, 19, 20, 62

   chronic, 132

   current medical view of, 62

   inherited, 15

   mental, 7, 14

   physical and psychological, 3, 14

immune system, 62, 63,

impact point(s),

   in brain, 39-40, 139, 140

   on left hemisphere, 143

   multiple, 140

indigestion, 240

influenza, 87, 117

META-

Diet, 228

Health, v- viii, xi, 3, 8-9, 16, 23, **25-45**, 90, 91,

analysis, vii, 39, 95-104, 117, 120, 124, 134, 221, 227-228

as an analytical tool, 9

approach, 187

coach, 134, 225, 229

concept, 79-80

Introductory Training, 95, 244, 246-249

model, 120, 154, 159, 214, 240

not a healing modality, 217

paradigm, 31

plan, 225, 229

practice, 94

principles, 3, 30, 115, 188, 190, 192, 207, 220-221, 226

meanings, 129

medicine, *see* META-Health

perspective, 10, 132, 188, 190-192, 225

position, 211, 214, 218-220

understanding, 32

metaphor, 166

metaphorical,

event, 37

interpretation, 52

microbes, 31, 76, 80

middle ear, 36

misperception(s), 58, 101

mood swings, 240

motives, misunderstanding, 151

movement,

issues, 97

theme, 36, 41, 56-57, 61, 146-148

mucous membrane(s)/mucosa, 71, 86, 176, 178

bladder, 107,126

bronchial, 38, 63, 70, 156-157, 163, 170, 222-223

larynx, 158

of nose, 125

rectum, 52, 148-149, 157

mucus, in stool, 52

multiple sclerosis (MS), 126

ovaries, 36, 85

ovarian cysts, 27

Overbruggen, Dr Rob van, xi, 6

oxygen, 68

P

pain, 18-19, 89, 98, 168, 209-10, 228

    abdominal, 118, 122

    coping with, 128

    during regeneration phase, 122

    lower back, 102, 112

    in lymph glands, 129

    musculo-skeletal, 118, 120-122, 129

    sensitivity to,

        increased, 126-127

        loss of, 131

palpitations, 118

pancreas, 84, 157

pancreatic duct mucosa, 86, 148-149, 157

parents, 54, 194

pelvis, 103

Pelzer, David, 210

perception(s), 37, 40, 50, 55, 56, **61-63**, 86, 97, 125, 135, 157, 166, 168

    changing, 139

    of danger, 22

    inherited, 93

    shift in, 163, 237

pericardium, 37, 85

peripheral vision, 71

peritoneum, 36, 61

personal development, 9

    tools, 214

perspective, 93, 106, 175, **189-190**, 209

    change/shift in, 10, 93

pharmaceutical companies, 80

pharyngeal tonsil (adenoid), enlargement of, 74

pharynx, 123-124

piles, 52

pituitary gland, 36, 62

placebo, 177

    effect, 43

pleura, 36, 85

positive thinking, 167, 183

post-traumatic stress disorder (PTSD), 117

practitioner, medical, 11

prostate, 36, 84, 141, 143

    cancer, 41

    enlarged, 144

protection, theme, 36, 41, 61, 95, 124, 144-146

protein(s), 43, 55

psychological,

    change, 139-154

    meaning, 221

Q

questioning techniques, 40, 101

quigong, Chinese health, 8, 228, 235

R

rage(s), 7, 151, 236

rash, 125

reaction(s), 50, 124

    allergic, 125

reality, creating, 187

recovery phase, 73

rectum, 36

    mucosa, 52, 148-149, 157

regeneration, 87, 88, 98, 127, 132, 174

    phase, 66, 73, 89, 99, 223

relationships, gay, 160

relaxation technique, 132

renal pelvis, 56, 59

repair, 27, 65-67, 76, 90, 91, 93, 120, 125, 127, 132

    activity, 82

    phase, 67, 68, 88, 93, 103

    process of, 67

reproduction, 41, 141

resilience, 16, 115, 225

resistance, subconscious, 198

resolution, 26, 52, 67, 72, 84, 89, 93, 98, 102-104, 174

    of original trauma, 87

    turning point, 99

response(s), 166-167, 212

    bio-logical, 37, 40, 91,154

    body, 68, 94, 166

    emotional, 190

    fight-or-flight, vi, 26, 61, 63, 65, 66, 71-72, 128, 132, 211, 236

    organ-tissue, 40

    patterns, 197

    to threat, 61

responsibility, 237

    individual, 221

reticular activating system (RAS), 207

reticular formation, 207,

retina, 86

    retinal vision, 71

tiredness, *see* fatigue

tissue(s), 55-57, 58, 220

    adaptation, 58, 93

    change in, 72, 139

    connective, 36

    fatty, 126

    functions, 48, 56, 60-61

    mammary, 75-76, 88

    normalisation, 90

    purpose, 222

    reaction, 120

    repair, 63, 73, 80

    response, 60, 136, 138

    strengthening/weakening, 61

    swelling, 102

    thinning, 61

tongue, 36

tooth,

    bone, 36

    enamel, 86

tonsil(s), 36, 73-75, 81, 82, 84, 87, 123

    tonsillitis, 75, 81

touch, sensitivity to, 131

toxin(s), 43, 206

transgender, 159

trauma, 9, 26, 38, 39, 40, 43, 48-49, 54, 56, 62, 67, 107, 110, 120, 124, 125, 133, 139, 143, 149, 151, 161-162, 184, 185-186, 209, 210

    of 'being thrown off course', 136

    emotional, 86

    of 'moving in wrong direction', 136

    perceived, 4

    physical, 43, 206

    processed, 164

    unprocessed, 201

    relating to the dis-ease, 137

    release, 69-70, 79, 189, **240-241**

        mechanism, 236

    traumatic event, 26, 48, 60, 67, 72, 83-84, 93, 136, 139, 153, 161, 171, 203, 224

    traumatic experience, 31, 38, 48, 73, 134, 149, 184, 220

About the author

S am is a META-Health Master Practitioner and Master Trainer. She delivers META-Health Introductory Training and Master Practitioner Training worldwide and is on the Advisory Board of the International META-Medicine Association.

With a background in teaching, Sam's greatest passion is delivering training. She also enjoys working as a consultant META-Health Coach and Energy Therapist, locally in Brighton and worldwide by means of Skype.

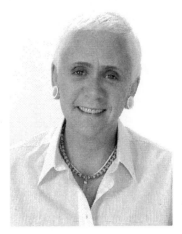

Sam Thorpe

Sam is an NLP Master, an AAMET EFT Practitioner Trainer and AMT Advanced EmoTrance and EFT Master Practitioner Trainer. She is also a trainer of EFT Picture Tapping Techniques and a qualified Chinese Health Qigong Instructor. Sam is also a qualified practitioner of Matrix Reimprinting using EFT, Matrix Birth Reimprinting, advanced PSYCH-K, Colour Mirrors, TRE – Trauma Release Exercises and is a HeartMath 1:1 and Group Provider.

More recently, Sam has been working together with her husband Vic, combining some of these advanced techniques with Vic's years of experience in the global workplace through their business 'IntoAlignment'.

Sam is creator and developer of the '7 Steps to Conscious Health™' personal breakthrough programme that includes her powerful stress and trauma processing technique 'Heart Alignment Process™' which you can read about in her new book: '7 Steps to Conscious Health - Believe in Your Power to Heal'. For more information about courses and professional training go to www.intoalignment.com

Printed in Great Britain
by Amazon

45959629R00167